Milady Standard
Razor Cutting
by Nick Arrojo

Milady Standard Razor Cutting by Nick Arrojo

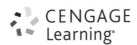

CENGAGE
Learning®

Australia • Brazil • Mexico • Singapore • United Kingdom • United States

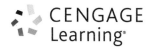

Milady Standard Razor Cutting
by Nick Arrojo

Executive Director, Milady: Sandra Bruce

Product Director: Corina Santoro

Product Manager: Philip I. Mandl

Associate Product Manager: Angela Sheehan

Product Assistant: Michelle Whitehead

Senior Director of Sales and Marketing:
Gerard McAvey

Marketing Manager: Elizabeth Bushey

Senior Production Director: Wendy Troeger

Production Director: Patty Stephan

Senior Content Project Manager:
Nina Tucciarelli

Senior Art Director: Benj Gleeksman

For product information and technology assistance, contact us at
Cengage Learning Customer & Sales Support, 1-800-354-9706

For permission to use material from this text or product,
submit all requests online at **www.cengage.com/permissions.**
Further permissions questions can be e-mailed to
permissionrequest@cengage.com

Library of Congress Control Number: 2014950279

ISBN: 978-1-2857-7807-5

Milady
20 Channel Center Street
Boston, MA 02210
USA

Cengage Learning is a leading provider of customized learning solutions with office locations around the globe, including Singapore, the United Kingdom, Australia, Mexico, Brazil, and Japan. Locate your local office at: **international.cengage.com/region**

Cengage Learning products are represented in Canada by Nelson Education, Ltd.

For your lifelong learning solutions, visit **www.milady.com**

Purchase any of our products at your local college store or at our preferred online store **www.cengagebrain.com**

Visit our corporate website at **cengage.com**

Notice to the Reader

Printed in the United States of America
Print Number: 01   Print Year: 2015

BRIEF CONTENTS

TABLE OF CONTENTS

ABOUT THE AUTHOR

Nick Arrojo's career began at Vidal Sassoon, Manchester, England. His talent for creative hairstyling was apparent early on, earning Nick the position of Vidal's youngest-ever Creative Director. He eventually moved to the United States, creating a multifaceted, multi-award-winning brand. Over a 30-year career, his work has graced the fashion magazines of the world on countless occasions while, as hairdressing host for seven seasons of TLC's *What Not to Wear*, Nick became an American household name. His beauty empire includes his NYC studio, a professional product line carried by hundreds of salons across America, and a cosmetology school and advanced academy that are both celebrated for their commitment to excellence, integrity, and raising the profile of the hairdressing craft. It is, however, Nick's pioneering method of modern and creative, precision-based razor cutting that draws the most acclaim. Taught around the world, his process enables hairstyles with the chic contemporary aesthetic of tapered edges and deconstructed textures. Nick lives in New York City with his wife Lina, and twin sons, Marco and Nico.

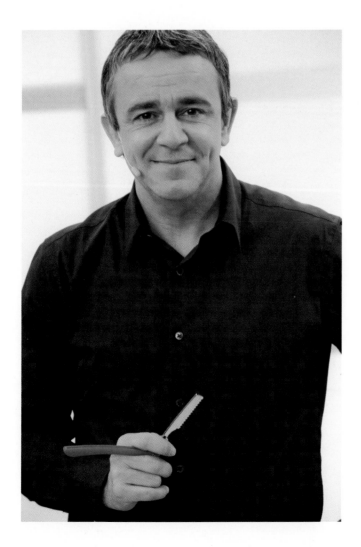

ACKNOWLEDGMENTS

A big thank you to all the people that worked on this project, especially Philip Mandl and Angela Sheehan from Milady, a part of Cengage Learning, and Andrew Arrojo.

To every person who picks up this book aspiring to be a better hairdresser, work hard, think big, and all your dreams will come true.

REVIEWERS

The author and publisher wish to acknowledge the following professionals for their support in the development of the manuscript by providing recommendations through their personal industry expertise.

Donna Charron, Eastern Wyoming College, Torrington, WY

Teresa Feltner, Rejoice Spa, Little Elm, TX

Michelle Richardson, Kenneth Shuler Schools of Cosmetology, West Columbia, SC

Betty Martinez, Houston Community College (Katy Campus), Houston, TX

Lynda Spittle, Scioto County Career Technical School, Lucasville, OH

Trudy L. Nicholson, Connellsville Area Career & Technical School, Connellsville, PA

INTRODUCTION

Welcome to my Milady Standard Razor Cutting workbook. Over six chapters, I am going to share my experience and expertise of this remarkable tool, giving you the elementary principles of proper use of the razor, so you can add a new range of techniques to your professional arsenal.

I believe you will find the razor perfect for shaping fashionable, low-maintenance modern hairstyles that your clients will love. Because the blade cuts length and weight at the same time, it empowers you to create tapered outlines naturally. Once you find a level of comfort using the tool, it becomes easier to put movement into styles, create more texture, and make beautiful, soft and fluid cuts.

To do these things well, you will need to develop an appreciation of the aesthetic differences of razor cutting, commit to mastering the technical fundamentals, and then have the passion and creative inspiration to want to develop your skills to the level of *a master*.

I begin the book with a look back at how the razor rose to prominence, and how its features and benefits match the fashion and beauty zeitgeist, creating conditions where proponents of razor cutting thrive.

Once the scene is set, I will show you the basics of contemporary razoring. From changing the blades safely to the all-important grip to moving and rotating the tool for a medley of effects, you will learn the fundamentals that go together to build a platform for success.

Then the fun really begins! Step by step by step, you will learn, practice, and master three razor hair cuts—the One-Length Bob with Blunt Bangs, Classic Long Layers with Choppy, Square Bangs, and The Bob with Graduation and Side-Swept Bangs—that give you an opportunity to implement the core skills of effective and artistic razor cutting.

In the nonfiction book, *Outliers: The Story of Success,* Malcolm Gladwell makes a compelling argument that the key to great accomplishments in any field is a matter of practicing a specific task for a total of 10,000 hours. It is something I wholeheartedly believe in; I was a hairdresser for 10 years before I began to feel like a master of the craft.

Please allow that thought to sink in. Realize that to become a master of razor cutting will take you many, many hours of practice. To make the most of this time, as you study the techniques in this book, I encourage you to scrutinize everything from body position and posture to the way I interact with the razor to how I carefully section the hair to how I focus on precise strokes and methodically check every section.

Soon enough, these techniques will become second nature to you, too, and you will begin to see the great potential of razor cutting to inspire ingenuity in your work, to make magic happen for your clients, and to become a signature of the success of your career.

HOW TO USE THIS BOOK

Performance Rubrics

At the end of each procedure, you will find a list of rubrics, or ways to note and comment on your performance for each of the key tasks. Rubrics are used in education for organizing and interpreting data gathered from observations of student performance. Rubrics are specifically developed scoring documents used to differentiate between levels of development in a specific skill, performance, or behavior. You can use rubrics to evaluate yourself, other stylists, and/or other students. As an instructor, you can use rubrics to evaluate your own students.

What's on the DVD?

To assist you in learning each and every step, the procedures can also be found on the companion DVD Series, *Milady Standard Razor Cutting with Nick Arrojo*. If you own this DVD or know that your school owns it, we encourage you to watch the procedure to strengthen your understanding of that particular procedure.

For more products serving practicing and future cosmetologists, please visit both www.milady.cengage.com and www.miladypro.com.

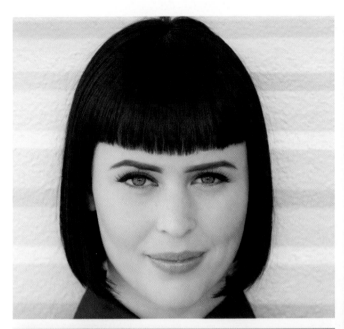

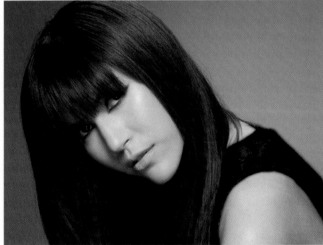

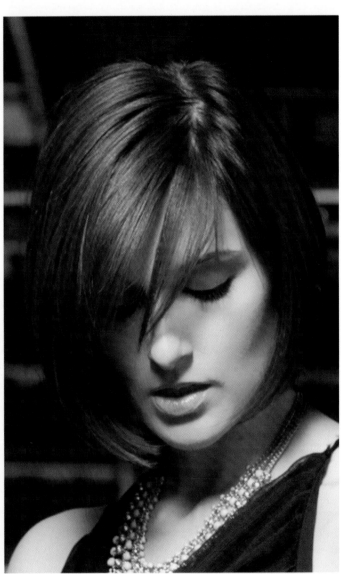

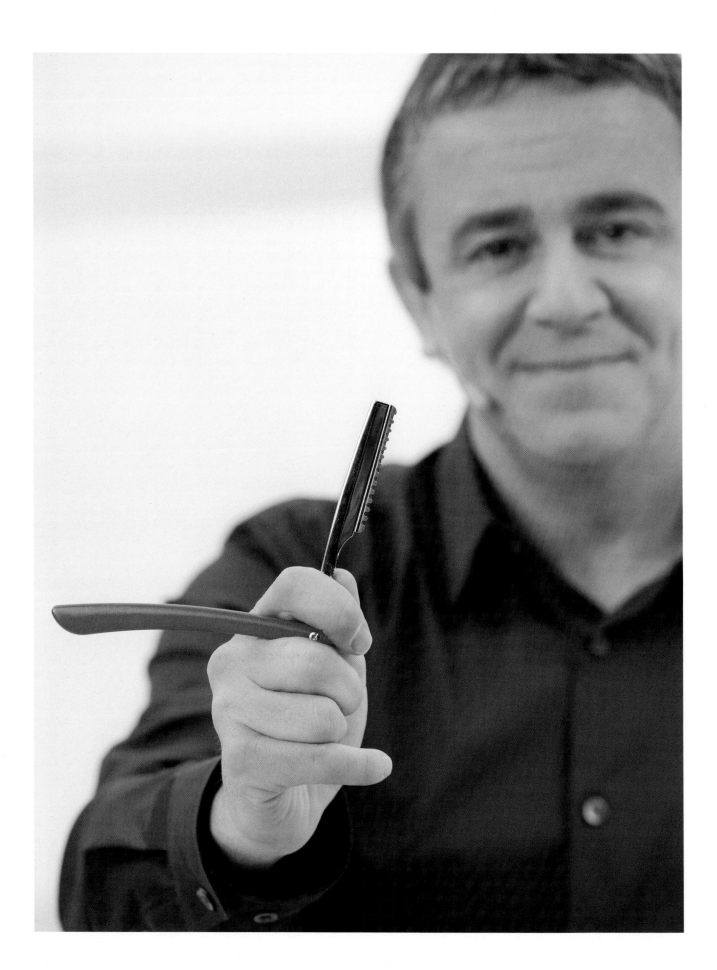

CHAPTER 1
THE RAZOR'S EDGE

Learning Objectives

After completing this chapter, you will be able to:

☑ LO❶ Recognize how and why fashion trends influenced a new direction for hairdressing.

☑ LO❷ Distinguish the key difference between shears and a razor.

☑ LO❸ Discuss how razor cutting can be a point of differentiation in your career.

INTRODUCTION: A BRIEF HISTORY OF RAZOR CUTTING

The first to champion the razor's use were the Japanese. Using their own traditional tools, and a technique named *Nihindo*, they found it a practical method for creating movement in straight hair. As a prelude to how it would become prominent in western styles, the Japanese realized that razoring was the best way to remove weight, to texturize, and to add movement. This was especially effective on the thick and straight strands that are indigenous to most people from this region. In the West, despite some brief periods of popularity, the razor only really gained traction as the new millennium approached. Even today, shears are most hairdresser's preferred method of cutting **(Figures 1-1 and 1-2)**.

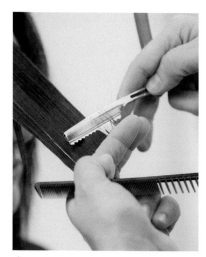

▲ **Figure 1-1** The tool and the techniques have evolved over time, but the inherent benefits of razor cutting remain the same.

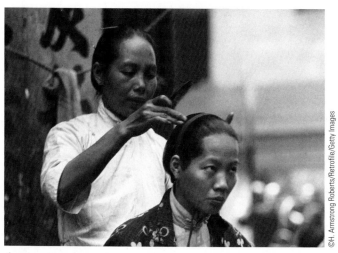

▲ **Figure 1-2** Asian culture has a longer, more consistent history of using the straightedge blade to cut hair.

LO ❶ Recognize how and why fashion trends influenced a new direction for hairdressing.

During the twentieth century, razor cutting came in and out of fashion. In the Roaring Twenties, Louise Brooks, siren of the silent film, embodied the daring spirit of the time with her trendsetting bob, cut with a razor. Her signature look featured heavy bangs, a tapered nape, and sleek points that enhanced her high cheekbones. Soon the bob was the dominant hairstyle in the western world as women who rejected traditional roles adopted the cut as a sign of modernity and freedom **(Figure 1-3)**. But as the 1930s dawned, so did an age of austerity, and fashion began to change. Women started to grow their hair longer, and the sharp lines of the bob were abandoned. Setting hair on rollers became popular; the art of the cut was out of favor. Shaped the same way in which canvas is cut to stretch and fit on a frame, from the 1930s to the 1960s, haircuts were made with the *styling*, not the *style*, in mind. Then came Vidal Sassoon. He pioneered a new direction for hairdressing, forged from his technical innovations. He treated hair like an architectural structure, not a piece of fabric. Using his shears to craft geometric, yet organic, shapes he was able to frame and complement the face without using elaborate and time-consuming hair-setting techniques. His far-reaching philosophy changed the approach of every stylist; even today, his influence is seen in haircuts from the runway to the street (**Figure 1-4**).

TAPERED EDGES BECOME FASHIONABLE

Vidal's vision of getting "down to the basic angles of cut and shape" created new, more efficient hairstyles that took over the world and made precision scissor-cutting the technique of choice. I became one of the disciples. My career began as an apprentice at Vidal Sassoon in the early 1980s. My education taught me the mastery of lines, layers, and graduation; the importance of precision; that craftsmanship and technique are the backbone of hairdressing. These things are as true today as they ever were. Then something happened that would begin to define my own career and the future of the craft.

By the late 1980s, I had become Vidal Sassoon's youngest Assistant Creative Director. As a prominent young stylist at the leading hairdressing brand in England, I was invited to style hair at London Fashion Week. One of the shows I was scheduled to work on was Ann Demeulemeester, the Belgium-born designer. I was so excited! Ann was part of a fashion circle that was known at the time as the *Antwerp Six*. The six designers from Antwerp's Royal Academy of Fine Arts had a reputation for a new type of fashion design, one that used precision craftsmanship to produce technically perfect tailoring. After construction, their garments were purposely pulled apart to create raw, frayed, tapered edges and beautiful silhouettes. The philosophy of the *Antwerp Six* was to deconstruct the traditional shapes and styles of fashion by using displaced seams and surface incisions. The results featured loose, elegant tailoring symbolized by the deconstruction in texture and "lived-in," perfectly imperfect feel.

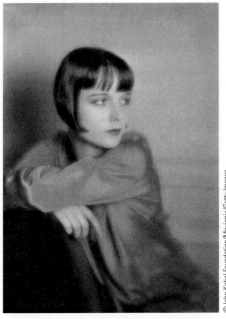

▲ **Figure 1-3** Louise Brooks's iconic razor cut from the 1920s.

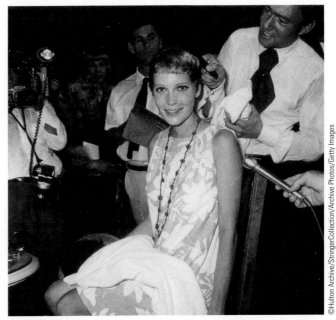

▲ **Figure 1-4** Vidal Sassoon cutting Mia Farrow's famous "crop".

WHY I MADE RAZOR CUTTING MY SIGNATURE TECHNIQUE

Thereafter, high street fashions started to show an influence from this avant-garde approach to tailoring. Although I continued to work to Vidal's original vision in the salon, in my own time I was now practicing using shears to create more than just geometry. I started to experiment with different ways of using my shears to create texture, movement, separation, and space. I was thinking about how to honor the outline of Vidal's architectural shapes, while deconstructing the interior. But I was frustrated at how much work I had to put in to soften the blunt edges of my scissor cuts; just to get close to the deconstructed effect I was looking for, I was manipulating my shears like a mad man!

Then I left Sassoon's for an opportunity to become the leading educator for Wella, United Kingdom. I was not working with clients in this new position, so it gave me freedom to practice and seek out the inspiration I needed to make the creative breakthrough I was looking for.

I traveled to Paris to meet Jean Louis David. I recall sitting with him on a boulevard in Paris, as he and I talked about the future of hairdressing. His career started in the 1960s, and Jean Louis became the French equivalent of Vidal Sassoon. He created his own techniques including the layer cut. He styled French movie stars and built an empire off of his skills. By the 1990s, his brand had stretched to New York where he opened a salon. I will always remember the essence of our conversation. He said that the next generation of pioneering hairdressers would need to blend the technical and artistic precision of Vidal Sassoon with the feel and the flair of the French, creating a new era of *"je ne sais quoi"* in hairdressing.

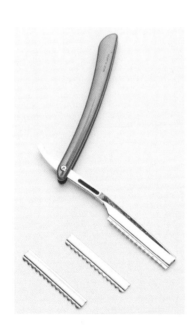

Jean Louis also spoke about razor cutting versus a classic scissor cut and how shears cut the ends bluntly, while a razor actually cuts into the hair, removing length and weight at the same time while also creating soft diffusion of texture instead of bluntness. It was not the first time I had thought about razor cutting, but after talking to Jean Louis and allowing my thoughts to percolate, I had clarity and inspiration. I was sure the *"je ne sais quoi"* was the razor. I got to work practicing all of Vidal's classic techniques, only this time cutting with a razor instead of shears, so I could see the natural difference of the two tools. As I began, my first realization was that I could actually feel the increased softness of the hair from the razor cut I was creating. As I cut, I felt more connected to the hair, and the razor felt like a more intuitive tool, with more freedom and creativity. I started to change the angle of the blade by using open and closed strokes, finding that I could make a blunt line if I wanted to, but that I could also use the razor to remove length and weight at the same time, while adding soft textural fluidity. I was creating classic shapes, as Vidal had done, but now I was able to deconstruct the interior, just as the Antwerp Six had done. The finished looks were softer and more versatile **(Figure 1-5)**.

In 1994, I was offered a new job in New York. I came to the Big Apple to accept the position of the Director of Education for Bumble and Bumble. At Bumble, I gained exposure to many of the modern world's best stylists. Their salon in New York brought together a global cast of masters of the craft who

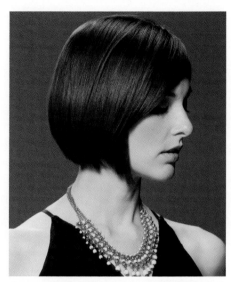

▲ **Figure 1-5** In a graduated razor cut, the hair blends together with a soft diffusion of texture.

fused techniques from all over the world with a special brand of creative expression and innovation. It was a joy to watch their virtuoso styles take shape. Noticeably, most of their work was done with a razor! This confirmed to me that razor cutting was becoming prominent, and it could potentially facilitate in my ability to put a signature on my talents. My thoughts were, "if one of the best salons on the planet was razor cutting hair, then other stylists would follow the trend, and I could become a leader for a pioneering new service and skill." Although my fellow stylists were creating some amazing work with their razors, I sensed the potential to do more. The features and benefits of the technique were just being discovered and were not yet mastered. I felt one of the issues was that the cuts were still being approached like an architectural structure. But I did not see it quite like that. I felt a connection to razor cutting because I saw something unique; I saw the opportunity to *carve out* the shape more intuitively. In short, I saw sculpture. I thought that if I could master how to "sculpt" hair with this tool, I could carve my niche in the industry, and maybe even help to shape how hairdressers in the future would go about their work **(Figure 1-6)**.

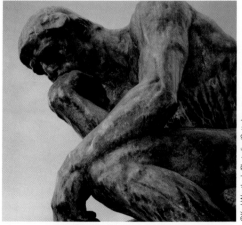

©Karl Weatherly/Photodisc/Getty Images

▲ **Figure 1-6** Razor cutting mirrors the artistic "carving out" of shapes that is found in sculpture.

A TOOL TAILORED TO FASHION-FORWARD CLIENTS

So I got busy honing and perfecting my technique. I found the razor to be an excellent way to create modern hairstyles. Creating swing and movement was so much easier. I began putting contemporary jagged lines into my cuts. Changing and tailoring texture was a cinch. I found a new love for short, messy, and shaggy styles. As for the soft-shaped layers, bam! **(Figure 1-7)**

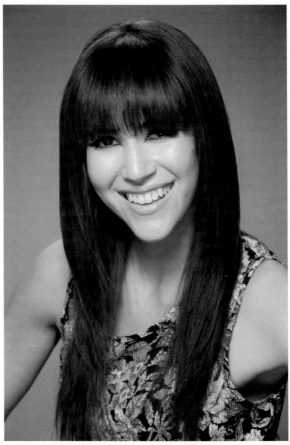

▲ **Figure 1-7** The layered razor cut is a classic modern style.

So it was not long before I felt confident enough to start using my new skills on clients. Happily, my hip, city-slicking clientele was as enamored with razor cuts as I was. As layers became weightless and curls sprang to life, as styles became moveable, touchable, and easy to style, more of my guests returned. Even better, they were bringing their friends!

A busy hairdresser is a successful hairdresser. I was able to build my "American Dream" upon the altar of my newfound skill. My experience taught me that the razor technique was perfectly suited to clients in the modern marketplace.

The subtle, yet pivotal, aesthetic differences of razor cutting have been discussed. There is no doubt that the soft, fluid lines, texture, and movement that influenced all avenues of fashion and design did play an essential part in evolving the preferences of trend-conscious clients. Something else was at work in these designs as well. The soft silhouettes combined with the loose, imperfect textures, in addition to the space and the freedom, were all conducive to *manageability*. With New York moving at such a fast pace, and working women balancing careers with personal lives, the days of idling away time with a blowdryer and a brush were fading fast. Women wanted and needed to "wash and go". I know this because hundreds, if not thousands, of clients have told me. It usually goes something like this: *"You know what I love most about my new style, Nick? All I have to do is towel dry, add in a bit of my favorite product, and that is it! I can run out the door, and I still get compliments!"* **(Figure 1-8)**

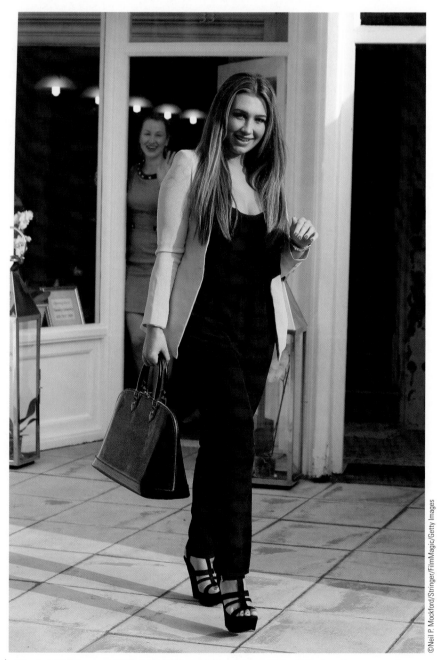

▲ **Figure 1-8** Make your clients look and feel great, and they will always be happy.

WHY THE RAZOR CAN TAKE YOU TO THE SHARP END OF SUCCESS

With all the positive experiences and feedback, I knew I was on to a good thing. Over the past 20 years, I have used razor cutting to underpin my success. My New York City Salon, ARROJO studio, is renowned all over the world for our signature techniques with the razor. I was even able to show the beauty of razor cutting to seven million weekly viewers on TLC's show, *What Not to Wear* (Figure 1-9). So with 20 years having passed since razor cutting started to show its teeth, one may think that cutting with a razor is the pre-eminent technique in hairstyling today. It is not. Trends trickle. Most top salons in big cities around the world are practicing razor cutting; but outside of the fashionable hubs, it is often an unknown or misused skill. I know this is true because I have also built a successful business in education. My team and I teach advanced classes to thousands of professionals across America each year. We also travel to all the major U.S. trade shows, which connects us to tens of thousands of stylists in just one place. One of the main skills we teach and champion is razor cutting. We find that some stylists are so inexperienced or unfamiliar with the tool that they perpetuate misguided ideas and beliefs and have little interest in learning more. Most do hold an interest in learning more, but many have a lack of knowledge and education, which means that they will need to take many classes and practice intently to become proficient.

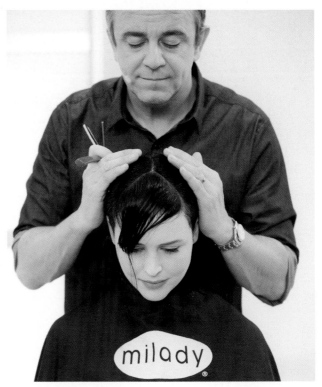

▲ **Figure 1-9** Nick Arrojo has become a world-renowned stylist based off of his signature razor cutting skills.

To cut right to it, razor cutting remains an elite practice. Not in an exclusive way; there is no band of stylists keeping it locked up because they only deem themselves good enough to use it, but in the way described, that only the top salons and stylists have taken the tool to heart. What an opportunity for you! If you take this tool to your heart, you immediately put yourself in the top 20 percent of hair stylists. Foremost, you will be a more rounded, progressive, creative, and versatile master of the craft. Then you will be a more attractive candidate for those top salons, which in turn, increases your earning potential because top salons are busier and have higher service prices. Next you will be dazzling that fashionable clientele with your cool, contemporary cuts. This preferred clientele is usually affluent, with many friends that they can recommend to you. As you become a veritable expert, you can be paid handsomely to teach other stylists what you now know: Mastery of a modern and creative, precision-based method of razor cutting makes magic happen for clients and for careers **(Figure 1-10)**.

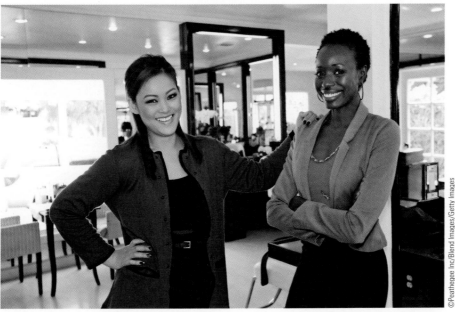

▲ **Figure 1-10** Adding razor cutting to your skill set increases your chances of a great career.

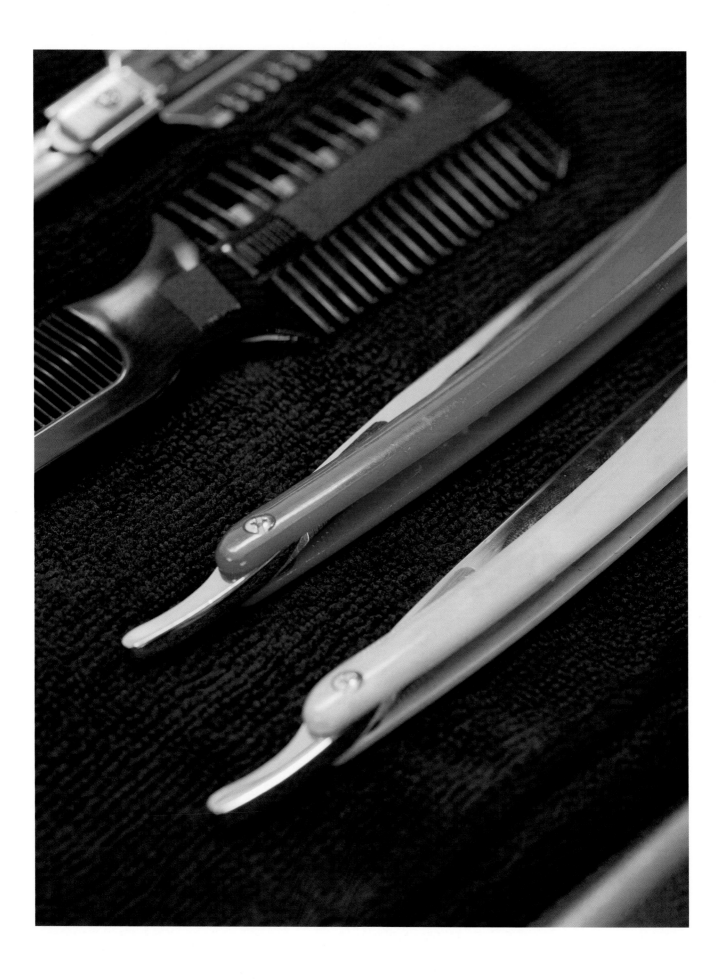

CHAPTER 2

BEFORE YOU BEGIN: THE KEY TENETS

Learning Objectives

After completing this chapter, you will be able to:

☑ ⃝ **❶** List the four golden rules of razor safety.

☑ ⃝ **❷** Cite the three key advantages to using a guarded razor.

☑ ⃝ **❸** Identify the anatomy of a razor.

☑ ⃝ **❹** List the steps on how to properly hold a razor.

☑ ⃝ **❺** Demonstrate how to comb and hold the hair in preparation for razor cutting.

☑ ⃝ **❻** Perform the proper razor cutting motion using the arm and shoulders; forearm; wrist and fingers.

☑ ⃝ **❼** Demonstrate the three core razor cutting techniques.

☑ ⃝ **❽** Demonstrate the steps on how to safely change the blades of a feather plier razor with detachable guards.

HEALTH AND SAFETY ALWAYS COME FIRST

Before getting excited about whipping out your razors, it is important to be aware of the possible dangerous situations you may encounter. Cutting yourself, a fellow stylist, staff member, or a client can do more than lacerate skin; it can break confidence in yourself, from your clients, and potentially peers. In the salon, the sight of blood is never good, especially in our world of beauty. As a beginner, I caution you to start out using a guarded razor as it is a lot less risky than the straightedge blade. While it still has the potential to cause injury, it is not nearly as bad. A guarded razor should help relieve any worry or nervousness you may have as you begin your razor cutting journey, not make you complacent.

Whenever I approach a razor cut, I imagine the razor as an extension of my mind's eye. I find how I handle and interact with the tool to be a critical part of the technique. So before we move on to the technical procedures and creative potential of razor cutting, we will examine how to handle and hold the razor, and the guarded blade, as well as how to safely change those blades. After we do that, I will show you how I like to interact with the hair as I razor cut and how I like to move and rotate the razor while I work, using a piston-like motion for smooth strokes and changing the angle of the blade for a range of creative effects. This is the beginning of your razor cutting journey. There are many exciting places it can take you.

Practicing the following safety routines will help to ensure no minor accidents while you master the tool. By the time you become more skilled, ready to take off the guard and work with a straightedge blade, your safety practices will be so ingrained that they will become second nature (**Figures 2-1 and 2-2**).

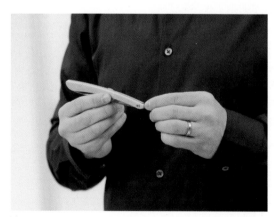

▲ **Figure 2-1** Even master stylists must take precautions when working with a tool as sharp as the straightedge razor.

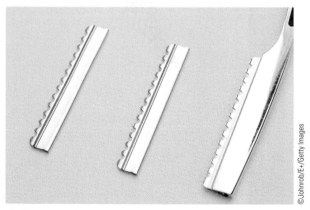

▲ **Figure 2-2** The guarded razor is the recommended tool of choice for beginners.

Accidents can happen at any time, but the good news is a simple commitment to vigilance and professionalism minimizes the risk, whether the blade used is guarded or not. Beginners should memorize and practice these four golden rules:

1. You must always be aware of where the razor is.

2. Make sure to close the razor anytime it is not in use.

3. Make sure the blades you are using have a guard attached.

4. While holding the razor, open or closed, always be aware of your body position and of what is around you.

These rules are easy to follow when picking up and putting away the tool, as there is not much else to distract you; but when you are working with a model or a client, and focused on your technique and creativity, while feeling the pressure to make the person in your chair happy, as well as having all the workings of a busy salon going on around you, it is easier for the brain to get muddled **(Figure 2-3)**.

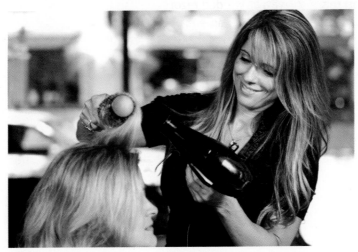

▲ **Figure 2-3** Be mindful of who and what is in your vicinity in the salon, as fellow stylists and their clients will usually be in close proximity.

Imagine for a moment that you have back-to-back clients on a busy and noisy day in the salon. Your first client arrived late, and your second arrived early. You are trying to perfect your first client's cut, while also being mindful of the time to not keep your second client waiting too long. The stylists that are working to your left and right are just as busy. With all this going on, you drop your comb as your prepare to razor cut your client's bangs. In this situation it would be easy to bend down to pick up your comb without thinking. This is where the dangers lie. With the razor blade open, you could cut yourself, your client, or a colleague. You must think first about where you are, where the razor is, and shutting the blade before doing anything else so the hazards are eliminated. The golden rules of cutting safely with a razor must be committed to mind and muscle memory. These rules should be memorized and practiced until they become an automatic trigger of your nervous system.

└○ ❷ **Cite the three key advantages to using a guarded razor.**

└○ ❸ **Identify the anatomy of a razor.**

HOW TO HANDLE AND HOLD THE RAZOR WITH THE GUARD

There are a couple of different types of razors available: stick razors **(Figure 2-4)** and electrical razor cutting combs **(Figure 2-5)**. However, these two tools may limit the ability to advance technique and creativity. Either of these two razor types

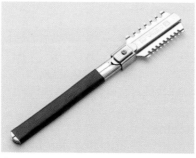

▲ **Figure 2-4** The stick razor.

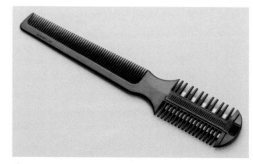

▲ **Figure 2-5** The razor cutting comb.

can be used when practicing the technical procedures in Chapters 3, 4, and 5, but due to their limitations, I highly recommend either a razor with pre-existing guarded blades or an unguarded feather plier razor with detachable guards. These two tools boast three key advantages:

1. You can practice safely with the guard on until comfortable with the tool and the techniques.

2. They have an ergonomic design that will provide the most versatility and creative freedom to move and rotate the blade.

3. The blade is the sharpest. This allows for precisely slicing through the hair and to tailor the effect of each stroke.

Handling and interacting with the razor is a critical part of the technique. To help you engage with the feather plier razor that is recommended, first examine its anatomy **(Figure 2-6)**.

Parts of the blade:

Front Edge: The first 1/3 inch (0.8 cm) of the front of the blade

Heel or **Back Edge:** The back 1/3 inch (0.8 cm) of the blade

Flat of the Blade: The width of the center of the blade

Once you are familiar with the tool, it is time to learn the all-important grip. Holding the tool properly enables a wider range of movements, aiding your creativity, while keeping you in control of the cut.

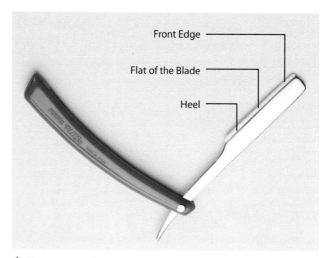

Front Edge

Flat of the Blade

Heel

▲ **Figure 2-6** The feather plier razor with detachable guards has three key elements to its anatomy: Front Edge; Heel; Flat of the Blade.

The proper way to hold the razor is in between the index finger and the middle finger, nice and tight. Your thumb should be placed on the groove of the grip and, with this snug fit, you should be able to make a wide range of motions, while keeping a level of control. One method to achieve the grip is as follows:

1. Begin with the handle on top and open the feather plier razor to a T-shape, with the blade facing up. The handle will be facing down toward the ground **(Figure 2-7)**.

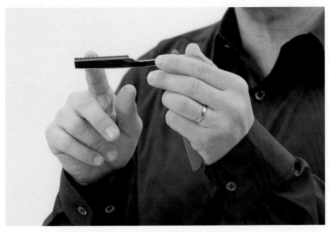

▲ **Figure 2-7** Open into a 'T' with blade up, handle down.

2. Turn your palm up, make a V for victory position with your index finger and middle finger, and slide the razor between these two fingers while resting your thumb on the grip. The guarded side of the blade faces you, and the open side of the blade faces the client. The open side of the blade makes contact with the hair **(Figure 2-8)**.

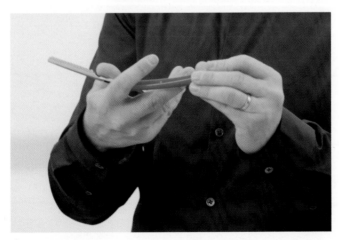

▲ **Figure 2-8** Rest your thumb on the grip for greater control.

3. Once you have your grip, you will notice that there is plenty of room between the blade and the thumb. This has dual benefits: one, this space makes it much more difficult to cut yourself; two, you still have three free fingers, which means you can comb and cut with the same hand, leaving

the other hand free for other work that may be required, such as holding and moving the hair as you cut (Figure 2-9).

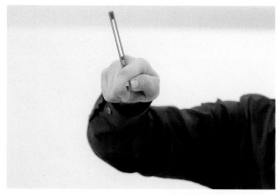

▲ **Figure 2-9** The blade should not be near the thumb.

4. Next try to wiggle your thumb. This is going to create control. It is going to engage the muscles of the index finger and middle finger to hold the blade steady so that the razor is not loose. Once you have practiced that, try rotating the thumb against the shaft of the blade, and wrap the pointer finger directly around the blade. Now take those fingers away, and leave the actual pointer finger wrapped around the blade. Look at where the tang is sitting: The tang sits right inside the palm of the hand. If this rotates out and comes through the fingers, it tells you that you are holding the razor incorrectly. So you want to always maintain a straight line as you hold the blade. We call this the lock and the load because the razor is locked in place (Figure 2-10).

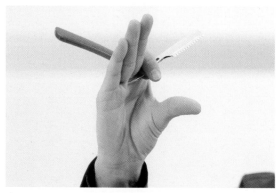

▲ **Figure 2-10** When in the lock and load position, it should be easy to move around your thumb and rotate the razor.

LO **8** Demonstrate the steps on how to safely change the blades of a feather plier razor with detachable guards.

CHANGING THE BLADES

Imagine slicing a tomato with a butter knife. The results would not be pretty. Do not expect that using a dull razor on hair will produce pretty results either. Please follow your state board guidelines in regards to how often you should change your blade and clean the body of the razor. Knowing the right way to safely change and store blades is important. Here is the procedure:

1. Carefully remove used blades by using a hard surface to push from the heel of the blade, moving the blade out. *Do not* pull the blade out using your fingers **(Figure 2-11)**.

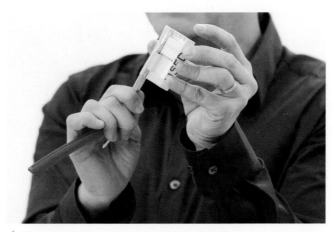

▲ **Figure 2-11** Always remove blades from the heel.

2. Handle the blade using the back, flat side to slide it into your razor blade container. Using a permanent marker, label dull razor blades so they are not used a second time. When the blade track is full, please also follow your state's guidelines on properly disposing of the used blades **(Figure 2-12)**.

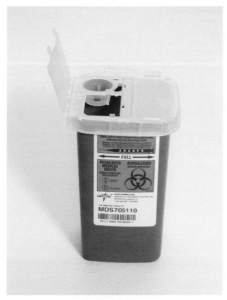

▲ **Figure 2-12** Organize and dispose of blades properly, like a professional.

3. Putting in a new blade is the same cautious process but in reverse: Again, using a hard surface for stability, push the blade in from the heel using the back, flat side to slide in the blade slowly and carefully. Ensure it is

properly secured, with the guard attached, and then close the razor until ready to use (Figure 2-13).

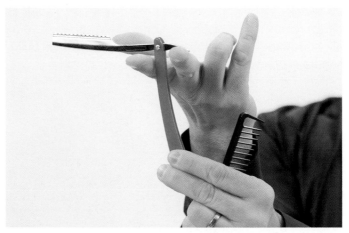

▲ **Figure 2-13** Always double-check that the blade is fitted securely before use.

LO **6** Perform the proper razor cutting motion using the arm and shoulders; forearm; wrist and fingers.

MOVING THE RAZOR

To begin cutting with the razor, never start from a motionless position. You need to use a smooth, piston-like motion that begins a few inches before reaching the hair. It is this fluid action that helps to slice through the hair effortlessly, creating beautiful texture. If you attempt to razor cut from a stiff position, your strokes will be ragged and so will the cut. The best advice for beginners is to keep the forearm and wrist almost perfectly still, and focus on making a mechanical arm motion, coming from the shoulder and the upper arm (Figure 2-14). This is a great way to impart smooth, back-and-forth movements with the razor. Once comfortable with this motion, you can begin loosening the forearm and wrist

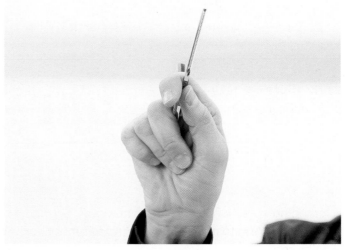

▲ **Figure 2-14** Imagine the smooth back and forth of a piston as your guide for your razor cutting motion.

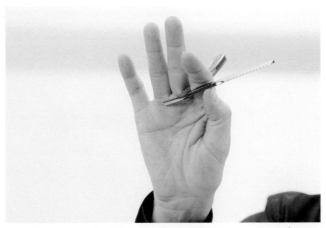

▲ **Figure 2-15** Using your forearm and wrist will widen the range of motions you can make while you work with a razor.

to achieve more flexibility and an increased range of movements **(Figure 2-15)**. After mastering that skill, the razor can be moved with just the fingers, while keeping the wrist, forearm, and shoulder as still as possible; once learned, this skill is the best way to achieve the most creativity and control **(Figure 2-16)**. Before doing anything else with a razor, recognize the importance of mastering the basic skill of even, fluid motion that starts before reaching the hair. To do so, practice all of these rhythmical movements in front of a mirror.

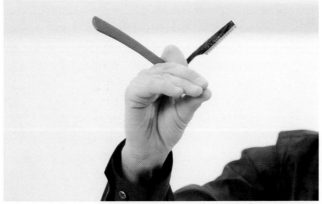

▲ **Figure 2-16** When you master smooth, piston-like movements, using your fingers, you have obtained the ability to create and control with maximum efficiency.

LO ⑤ **Demonstrate how to comb and hold the hair in preparation for razor cutting.**

HOW TO HOLD HAIR FOR PERFECT RAZOR CUTS

Whenever prepping a section of hair for a razor cut, the first step is using the fine teeth of the comb to maintain good, strong tension for cutting. After which, the main consideration is how to hold the hair for the razor cut. Unlike with shears, where often the comb is used to hold hair in place as you cut, with a razor, always use the fingers––for control and versatility. The technique is as follows:

1. Comb the hair with the fine teeth of the comb. Ensure strong, even tension on each section about to be cut **(Figure 2-17)**.

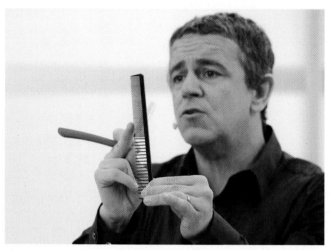

▲ **Figure 2-17** Use the fine teeth of the comb to create tension for cutting.

2. As the comb comes down and through the hair, follow the path with your non-dominant (non-cutting) hand. Once the comb has created the tension you want and has reached the ends of the hair, place the hair in between the index finger and middle finger using your non-dominant hand, keeping the fingers horizontal **(Figure 2-18)**. When it comes to razor cutting, you have got to make sure that you get the hair really taut and really tight, so focus on maintaining tautness as you place the hair between your fingers.

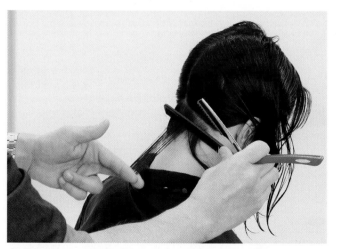

▲ **Figure 2-18** Use both the index finger and middle finger for holding hair securely with strong tension.

3. Remember that when you are cutting with a razor, you are cutting into the hair and not just the ends of the hair, which is what you would do with shears. As you cut, you must slide your index finger and middle finger down the hair shaft, while maintaining even tension **(Figure 2-19)**.

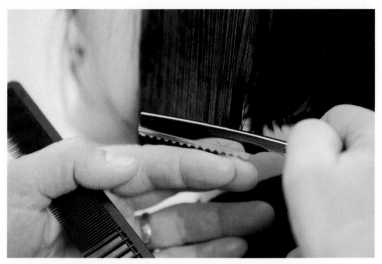

▲ **Figure 2-19** Learn to slide fingers through hair while maintaining tension.

RAZOR AEROBICS

When I was teaching myself razor cutting, I developed a procedure I like to call *Razorobics.* The idea is to put the repetitive actions of razor cutting into your muscle memory. In front of a mirror, practice all the movements we have discussed, from taking your grip to the lock and the load to the comb and the cut. To begin, have the razor closed. Now, open it to a T, make your V for victory position with your fingers, and take your grip. Now place the comb in your three free fingers, creating the lock and the load. Imagine you have a client sitting in a chair in front of you. Slowly at first, complete the actions of the razor cut: section; rotate; comb; hold; place; cut. And repeat: section; rotate; comb; hold; place; cut. Keep speeding it up until you are a master of razor aerobics **(Figures 2-20 and 2-21)**.

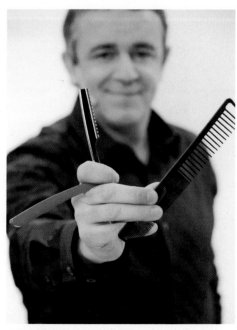

▲ **Figure 2-20** The lock and the load position is the starting point of razor aerobics.

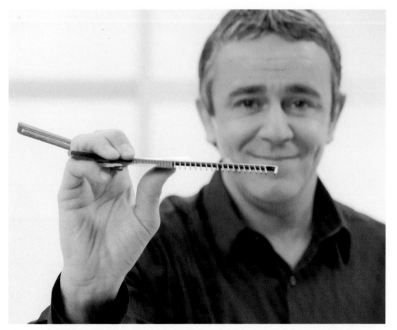

▲ **Figure 2-21** Learning to safely and precisely move and rotate the comb is one of the key benefits of practicing razor aerobics.

THE ANGLE OF THE BLADE: DIFFERENT USES, FEATURES, AND BENEFITS

Once you are familiar with the razor, have learned the basic technique for moving the razor back and forth like a piston, and have achieved the skill in handling and holding the hair as you cut, you can begin to expand your skill set. One of the best aspects about razor cutting hair is versatility. Even the smallest rotations of the blade make a big difference.

The most common razor technique is *closed blade*. Cutting with a closed blade comes closest to the effect of a shear-cut, but with much more softness and texture. You will use this technique for one-length razor cuts, as this technique is perfect for blunt lines, strong outlines, and the most amount of weight. When using this skill, use short methodical strokes **(Figure 2-22)**.

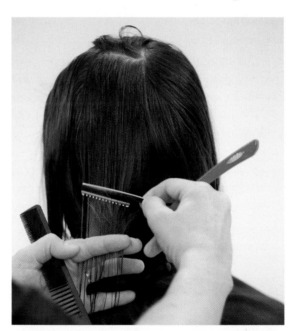

▲ **Figure 2-22** The closed-blade razor cutting technique features slow, smooth, and systematic strokes.

The other main razor technique is *open blade*. Cutting with an open blade creates texture, removes length and weight at the same time, diffuses the ends into a finer and softer style, and adds space. This helps the hair to swing and move. Most often, this technique is used on graduated and layered shapes. Creative short shapes are also created using open-blade cutting. The more you open the blade, the more you texturize the hair **(Figure 2-23)**.

Another type of razor technique is called *tipping out the weight*. This skill is mainly used for refining the finished cut with a creative touch. Tipping out the weight is a texturizing technique that creates space in the hair by using the front edge of the razor. It is not used when cutting more than 2 inches (5 cm) deep from the ends of the hair. It can be used in one of two ways: vertical or horizontal. Vertical tipping out the weight removes less weight and is great for

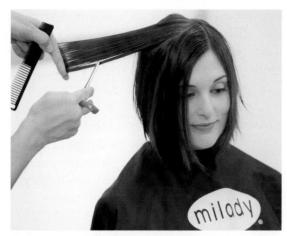

▲ **Figure 2-23** Using an open blade is a creative technique for removing length and weight; practice opening the blade to different degrees to see and feel the effects.

a seamless, smooth surface. Horizontal tipping out the weight removes the most weight, creates the most space, and creates the most texture. With an unguarded razor, the very tip of the blade is used, as the closer to the tip, the stronger the effect. However, when using a guarded razor this technique comes with a limitation. The guard of the razor covers the very tip, so this skill would need to be practiced by using the first corrugated edge of the guard. It is not quite the same effect as using the very tip of an unguarded razor, but you will see the benefits of the technique **(Figure 2-24)**.

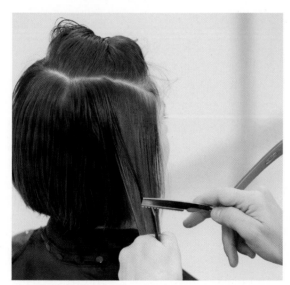

▲ **Figure 2-24** Practice tipping out the weight with your guarded razor; by the time you are ready to take the guard off, you willbe an expert exponent of this advanced technique.

RESULTS OF DIFFERENT HAIR TYPES

There are many people that misconstrue what a razor can and cannot do. I have had clients come to me and tell me, *"I got a razor cut after seeing some of the work you have done with the tool, but look what it did to my hair. It is in tatters."* This is not limited to salon guests. I have also heard experienced professionals say: *"Do not get your hair cut with a razor; the wreckage is too hard to repair."* Erroneous assumptions stem from a lack of knowledge. Razor cutting education is harder to find than classic-cutting education, hair-coloring education, and permanent-texture education. Like anything else in this world, when there is an education gap, inaccurate ideas flourish. Razor cutting's most in bloom misconception is the idea that certain hair types, typically fine or curly textures, are not suitable for razor cuts. From this, all sorts of untruths have cropped up; let us clear a few of them up.

On fine hair, the razor is actually better than shears. The blunt lines of a shear cut are unforgiving, as they reveal just how fine the hair is. Conversely, when cut with a razor, the diffused, tapered edges will blend and disguise the fineness of the texture, which is much better for the hair and the style.

With wavy and curly hair, there are some challenges to overcome. Specifically, stylists need to be careful not to put too much texture into hair that is already textured; they need to be careful not to take out too much weight because density often helps the structural integrity of curls; and they need to be careful not to "thin out" the hair too much as this can make curls fall flat. Since the razor is a tool that naturally does all of the above (texturize, remove weight, thin-out), and it takes experience to know when and how to tailor the approach to different textures, it is not surprising to see inexperienced razor cutters give the straightedge blade a bad name when they choose to use it on curly hair.

What we must remember is that, employed correctly, the razor can be used for almost anything a stylist will want to achieve in their hair cutting. It can cut only length, add weight, and make blunt lines. The razor is capable of doing what your shears do, and it is also more versatile. Once you become proficient, you may find, like me, that on curly hair, you can do more intricate work with a single blade than anything you could accomplish with shears. Contrary to the myth, a master razor cutter cuts beautiful curls filled with body and bounce **(Figure 2-25)**.

Perhaps the only hair type to avoid razor cutting is highly textured, coarse, and coily hair. Due to the coarseness of the strands, they tend to shred when

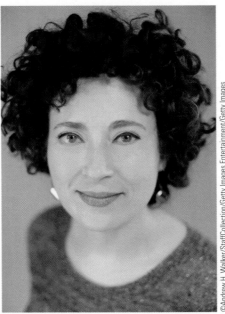

▲ **Figure 2-25** Razor cut curls can and should be beautiful.

they meet the blade. This makes it difficult to create a consistent cut. Since the level of coarseness varies from person to person, this is not a golden rule. Similar to a strand test performed when chemically treating the hair, you can cut a few strands with the razor first, to test how the hair will react. If the ends do not shred, it is a sign a razor cut will be fine. However, if the shredding is bad, switch to shears.

Another myth is razor haircuts cause hair to be frizzy, when the truth is they do not. Whatever the tool, too much texturizing or too much thinning out of the hair can make a hairstyle prone to frizz. Since the razor is often used for weight removal, taking out weight, and adding texture, it means that someone who is inexperienced with the tool and the techniques may undermine the benefits of the straightedge blade with heavy-handed work that creates frizz for their clients. A proficient exponent of this art, on the other hand, understands when and how to add texture or remove weight, and will focus more on creating shapes and styles with tapered edges, softness, movement, and fluidity––the key advantages of razor cutting.

TALKING TO CLIENTS ABOUT THE RAZOR CUT

With the false impressions of razor cutting clients might already have, there will be times when you deem using a razor technique to be ideal, only for the client to be concerned about the results. As a professional, it is your responsibility to make the person in your chair feel excited and confident. For that to happen, you have to be experienced and confident in your skills, both technical and verbal. Communication skills are critical. A seasoned stylist is almost always a great communicator, so this is a chance to practice an important part of your job. If you can ease the client to earning your trust, chances are that that is a client for life **(Figure 2-26)**.

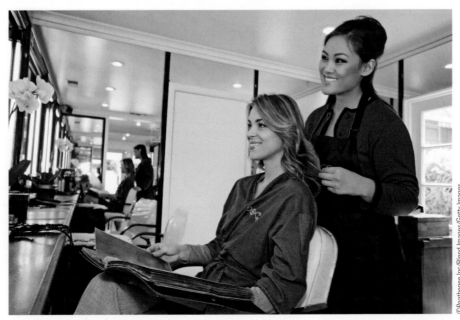

▲ **Figure 2-26** Mastering technical skills is only half of your job; effective client communication is what separates the great from the good.

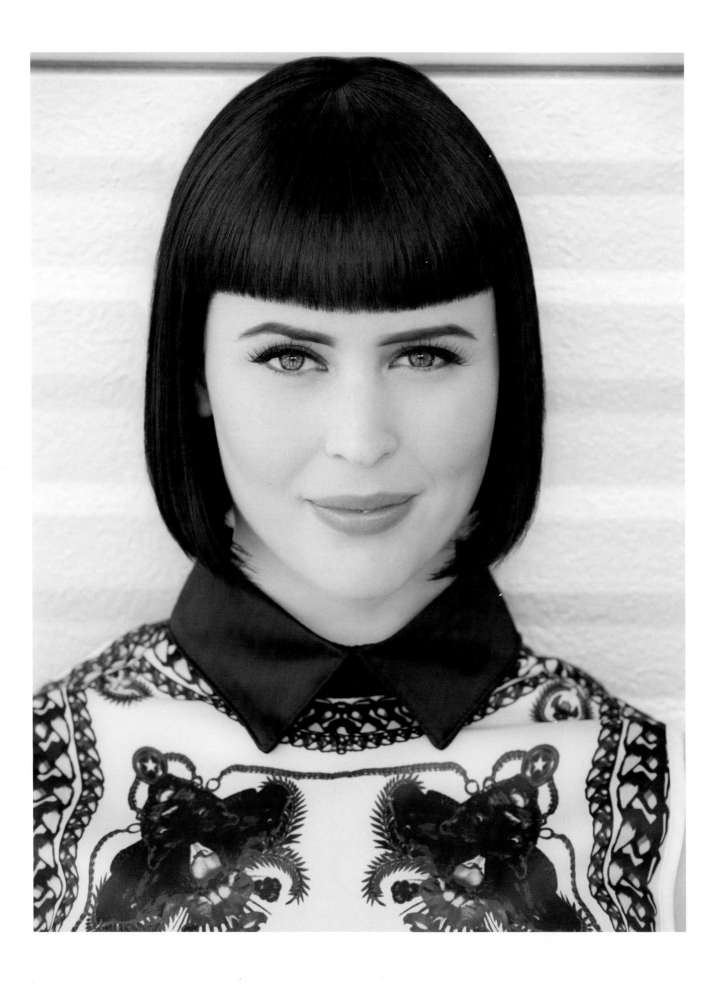

CHAPTER 3
RAZORING A ONE-LENGTH LINE

Learning Objectives

After completing this chapter, you will be able to:

☑ LO❶   Execute the correct sectioning patterns for this haircut.

☑ LO❷   Demonstrate how to create the first section as a guideline for the rest of the haircut.

☑ LO❸   Demonstrate combing the hair with even, consistent tension.

☑ LO❹   Perform a piston-like razor cutting motion while using the closed blade technique.

☑ LO❺   Demonstrate how to check for balance and how to refine if necessary.

☑ LO❻   Demonstrate ability to cut both sides with perfect balance.

☑ LO❼   Execute blunt, square bangs.

THE ONE-LENGTH BOB WITH BLUNT BANGS

Expertly cut, the classic one-length bob with blunt bangs fashions a sophisticated, poised, and polished style. Featuring the timeless elegance, beauty, and grace of a clean line, hair is razored without any layers or graduation to maintain a solid outline: 0-degree elevation to create maximum weight. After completion, hair should sit above the shoulders but below the hairline at the nape. It is important to use the closed-blade razor cutting technique. To produce the blunt lines synonymous with this cut, the blade must go through hair at a 90-degree angle. The beauty of practicing this style with a guarded razor is the opportunity to give a modern twist to a classic shape. The blade naturally creates a diffused, tapered outline, which gives the cut a contemporary, streamlined, and chic look. As the style increases the appearance of weight, it is ideal for anyone with fine hair texture. The cut is also perfectly suited to any client with straight to slightly wavy, sleek, and healthy hair. For you the stylist, conquering one-length haircutting is a key part of your journey to mastery of the craft. Learn this technique and one of the pivotal fundamentals will be in your locker forever, always ready for the right client, at the right time.

IMPLEMENTS AND MATERIALS

You will need all of the following implements, materials, and supplies:

- Cutting cape
- Guarded razor
- Neck strip
- Sectioning clips
- Spray bottle with water
- Towels
- Wide-tooth comb
- Blowdryer
- Oval flat brush

HERE'S A **TIP:**

Ensure the client is sitting straight (arms and legs uncrossed) so that the body is not off-balance. If the client is sitting off-balance, it may affect the quality of your line.

PROCEDURE: The One-Length Bob with Blunt Bangs

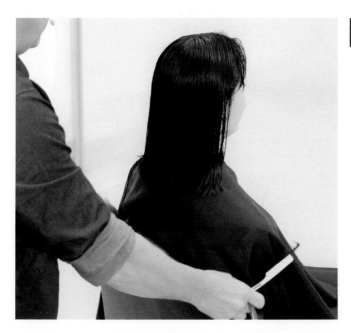

1 Position the client carefully in the chair. The client's head should be parallel to your chest level.

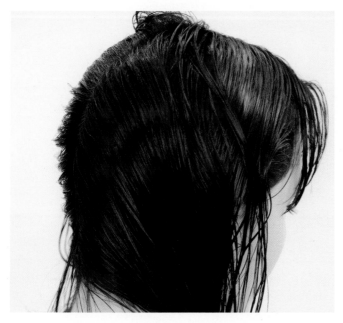

2 Next, using your sectioning comb, create a center part from the forehead to the nape.

PROCEDURE: The One-Length Bob with Blunt Bangs

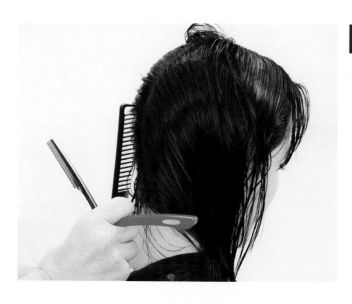

3 At the nape, create a ½-inch (1.25-cm), slight diagonal subsection that mimics the arch of the neck. Divide this first section in half.

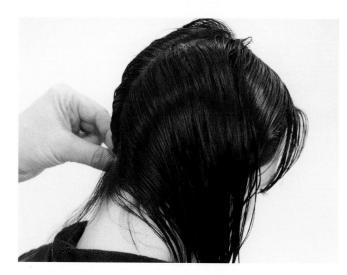

4 Tilt the client's head slightly forward so that the body position is at its most natural. This flattens out the back of the neck, giving you a level surface to work on, which helps you to prevent graduation in the line.

HERE'S A **TIP:**

As is always the case with the guarded razor, you will start from the center back and work from side to side as you move up the back of the head; this is the best way to create consistency.

PROCEDURE: The One-Length Bob with Blunt Bangs

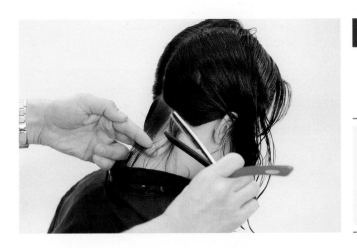

5 Position yourself directly behind the client, parallel to the nape. You will need to move slightly from side to side to cut each side of the back section. At the nape, create a half-inch, slight diagonal subsection that mimics the arch of the neck. Divide this first section in half.

HERE'S A **TIP:**

Concentrate on using no elevation or over direction as you section. It is critical; otherwise you will create graduation in the shape.

HERE'S A **TIP:**

Remember, you are cutting across the hairline at the back of the neck; a square bob line at the nape will have the appearance of a very slight arch, just as the neck does. Because of this, make your sections on a slight diagonal—not quite horizontal, not quite diagonal, but in between, so that it mimics your cutting line on the nape.

6 Using your comb, create half-inch thick sections of hair.

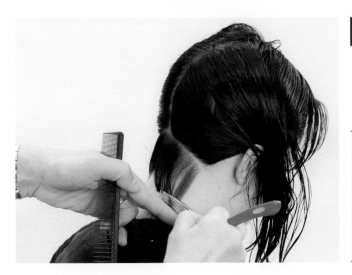

7 Using a closed-blade technique, cut to the desired length with a square line, tight tension, and 0-degree elevation on both sides of the first section.

HERE'S A **TIP:**

Once you have cut your first section, you have created your guide. Two points here: One, the first section is critical because that is the guide that you will follow. Two, always follow that guide.

PROCEDURE: The One-Length Bob with Blunt Bangs

8 Using the first section as your guideline, continue working up the back of the head, taking ½-inch (1.25-cm) sections; complete both sides of each section before dropping down the next section. ☑ LO ❷

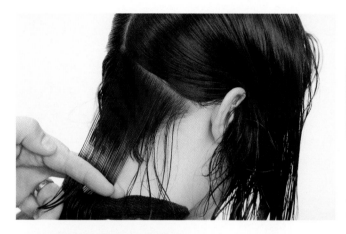

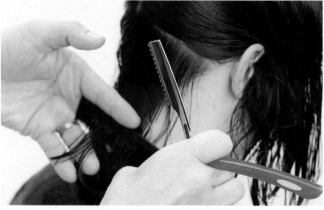

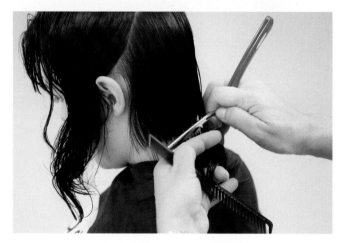

HERE'S A **TIP:**

Be mindful that the sections of hair that you pick up to cut are not too thick not too thin. Half-inch sections should be your goal. Most importantly, all sections should be of even, consistent size.

PROCEDURE: The One-Length Bob with Blunt Bangs

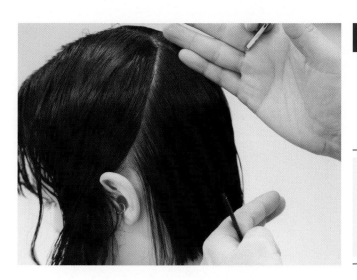

9 After cutting three sections on both sides of the back of the head, check the balance. Ensure you have a clean, square line before dropping down the next section. As you work up the head, consistency between the sections from the nape up to the occipital bone and the drop back crown should be checked often.

HERE'S A **TIP:**

When cutting a one-length line, always keep your eye on the prize. The prize is the one-length baseline at the back. Make sure it is always kept solid and straight and smooth.

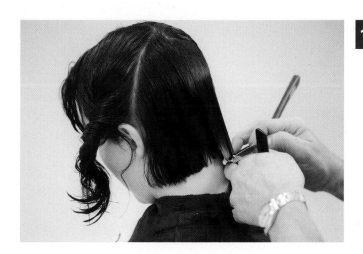

10 Continue working is consistent sections up to the occipital bone.

PROCEDURE: The One-Length Bob with Blunt Bangs

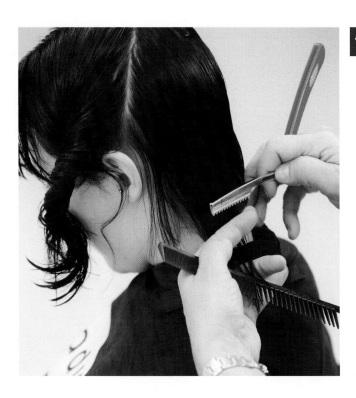

11 As you cut through the sections, comb hair side to side to encourage the visual turning under of hair, which will enable you to see the style falling into place.

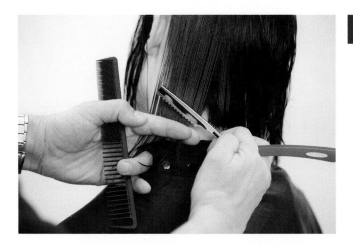

12 As you move up the head to complete the sections in the back, the sections will rotate, staying behind the back of the ear. Create a diagonal section from the crown to behind the ear, and cut to the desired length with a square line, even tension, and 0-degree elevation. Complete this section on both sides of the head.

PROCEDURE: The One-Length Bob with Blunt Bangs

13 Once the back sections have been cut cleanly and precisely, it is time to move to the sides. To cut the sides, take a swooping section all the way from the center back so it is parallel to the exterior shape. Using the fine teeth of the sectioning comb, divide the hair behind the ear.

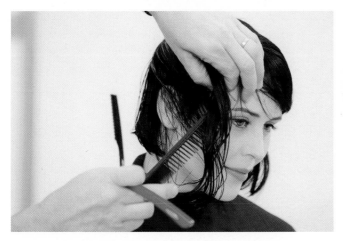

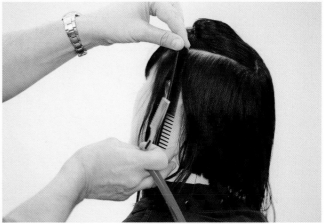

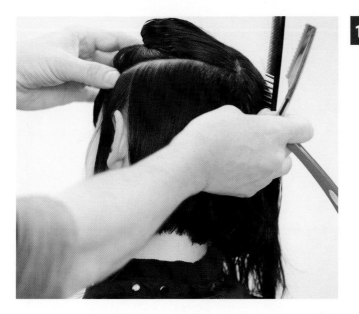

14 Before you begin, position the client's head upright and slightly tilted away from you.

PROCEDURE: The One-Length Bob with Blunt Bangs

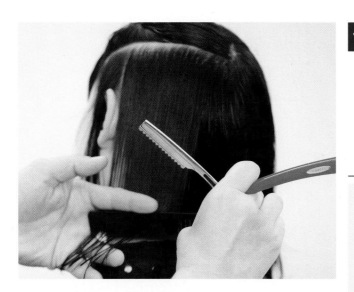

15 To successfully cut the side sections, you must continue your line from the back. Once you have established your guideline from the back, comb the side section down, using the narrow teeth of the comb to maintain tension with no elevation or over direction. When combing the side sections, be mindful of the ear. The ear is a small obstacle in your path, so good, consistent, strong tension will help you to smoothly comb hair over this area as you maintain a clean line.
☑LO❸

HERE'S A **TIP:**

Always keep hair evenly saturated. If hair is too dry when you razor cut it, you will create snags and tears; if hair is too wet, hair becomes uncomfortable to handle and hard to control. A good test: Hair should be wet to the touch, but not dripping wet. Always have a water spray bottle at hand.

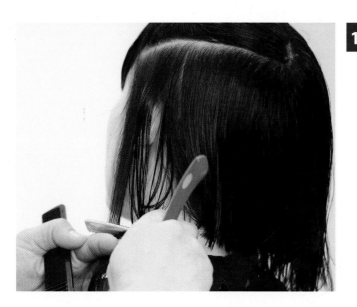

16 Secure hair between the index finger and middle finger (as outlined in the How to Hold Hair for the Perfect Razor Cut section of Chapter 2.) and, using the previously cut back section as a guide, continue cutting the back side to the back of the ear.
☑LO❹

PROCEDURE: The One-Length Bob with Blunt Bangs

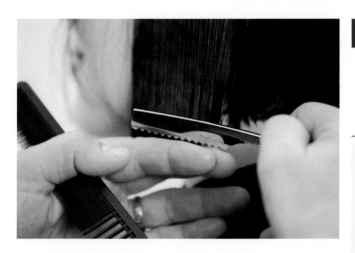

17 Continue to check that you are following your guide and cutting the desired angle as you work in half-inch sections up the head until you reach the center-parting. As with the back, monitor that you are maintaining 0-degree elevation and good, even, comb tension throughout. Ensure you have a clean, square, well-balanced line before dropping down the next section.

HERE'S A **TIP:**

Unlike cutting with shears, where hairlines, growth patterns, and head contours may change your approach, razor cutting is all about cutting with the right tension. Do not concern yourself with hairline issues; focus on cutting precision sections with good, consistent tension. Any problems related to the hairline should be corrected after blowdrying.

18 Move to the opposite side, and repeat steps 14-18. Remember to keep the client's head upright and tilted slightly away from you. Check both sides for balance before completing this side, and refine as necessary.

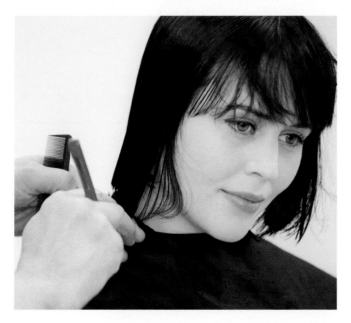

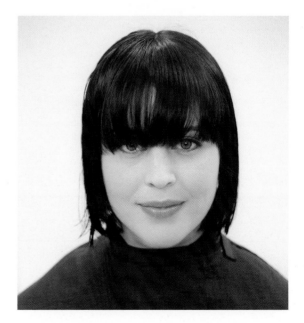

PROCEDURE: The One-Length Bob with Blunt Bangs

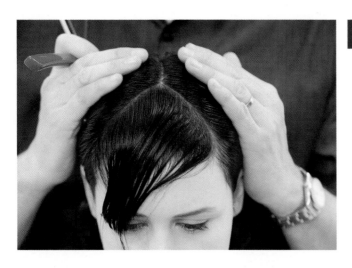

19 To create square bangs to match this one-length style, start by creating your bang section. Make a triangular-shaped section from the top of the center parting to the recession. This ensures that the bangs will fall naturally into place, wide of the eyes.

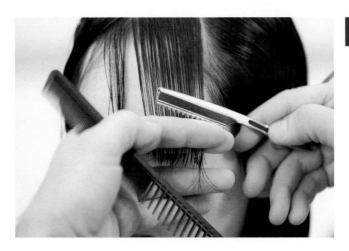

20 Begin the bang cut by taking a section from the outside corner of the triangle, where it meets the recession. Comb this section straight down and cut a square line to the desired length, just above the eyebrow. From the same side, working up and along the triangle until you reach the central parting, make and cut two more sections in exactly the same fashion: Comb each section straight down, and cut a square line to the desired length. Then move to the opposite side of your original triangle, and repeat this step.

PROCEDURE: The One-Length Bob with Blunt Bangs

21 Once all sections of the triangle are cut, comb the whole-bang section forward to check length and weight. Refine if necessary.

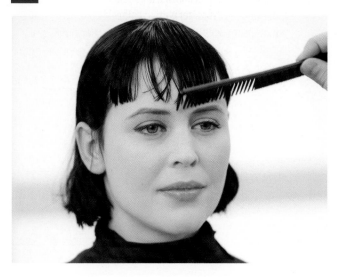

☑ LO❺
☑ LO❻
☑ LO❼

HERE'S A **TIP:**

Mastering this cut will give you the fundamentals of cutting all one-length hair, which is one of the key techniques of great stylists.

22 To do a beautiful, swinging blowdry, you are going to wrap the hair around the head, using the surface of the scalp and a flat paddle brush to blowdry the hair nice and smooth, and with consistent root lift, until it is close to dry.

PROCEDURE: The One-Length Bob with Blunt Bangs

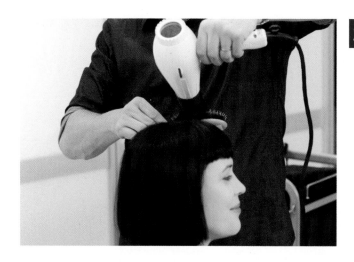

23 With the hair now 75-85% dry, apply some thickening lotion, and section hair by mimicking your cutting sections. Start at the nape, and blowdry with a flat paddle brush. Dry from roots to ends taking one-inch sections, working up the head. Blowdry with only a little root lift and, vitally, make sure the amount of root lift is consistent throughout. Otherwise, the integrity of the finished style can be compromised which makes it more difficult to properly clean and check your one-length line.

24 Make sure that each section is completely dry before proceeding to the next one.

25 When approaching the ends, a slight inward bending will complete the style with a chic finish.

PERFORMANCE RUBRICS

The following rubrics are used for organizing and interpreting data gathered from observations of performance regarding this one-length guarded-razor haircut. It is a clearly developed scoring document used to differentiate between levels of development in a specific skill or behavior. I recommend they be used as a tool to gauge progress, either through self-assessment or with the aid of your educator. Write down your notes, chart the development of your skills, and vow to never stop learning.

Performance is evaluated according to the following scale:

1. **Development Opportunity:** There is little or no evidence of competency; Assistance is needed; Performance includes multiple errors.
2. **Fundamental:** There is beginning evidence of competency; Task is completed alone; Performance includes few errors.
3. **Competent:** There is detailed and consistent evidence of competency; Task is completed alone; Performance includes rare errors.
4. **Strength:** There is detailed evidence of highly creative, inventive, mature presence of competency. Space is provided for comments to assist you in improving your performance and achieving a higher rating.

Performance Assessed	1	2	3	4	Improvement Plan
Demonstrated correct client body positioning in chair					
Demonstrated correct sectioning technique in the back sections					
Demonstrated correct way to tilt client's head for razoring back sections					
Demonstrated correct amount of hair to cut in each section (half-inch)					
Demonstrated correct amount of comb tension					
Demonstrated 0-degree elevation while combing hair in preparation for the cut					
Demonstrated ability to cut to desired length in a square line					
Demonstrated ability to create even, consistent sections from the nape to the drop back crown					
Demonstrated ability to use first section as guide for the rest of the cut					

Performance Assessed	1	2	3	4	Improvement Plan
Demonstrated ability to check sections visually as well as technically					
Demonstrated correct sectioning pattern for cutting the side sections, including how to continue the guide line from the back					
Demonstrated correct procedure for combing over ear with even, clean tension					
Demonstrated ability to work up the sides in half-inch sections while maintaining 0-degree elevation					
Demonstrated ability to cut both sides with perfect balance					
Demonstrated ability to cross-check each side using a mirror for a side-by-side comparison					
Demonstrated ability to check finished cut reaches desired length and is a squarely angled one-length line					
Demonstrated correct sectioning pattern (triangle) for blunt bangs					
Demonstrated correct procedure for razoring bangs in a square line to desired length					
Demonstrated correct blowdry procedure					
Demonstrated ability to properly check and, if necessary, refine finished one-length style					
Demonstrated ability to hold the hair in hands correctly in preparation for razoring (see Chapter 2 for thorough explanation of the technique). This should be maintained throughout the entire procedure.					
Demonstrated ability to use a piston-like movement while razoring with a closed blade (see Chapter 2 for thorough explanation of the technique). This should be maintained throughout the entire procedure.					

FRONT

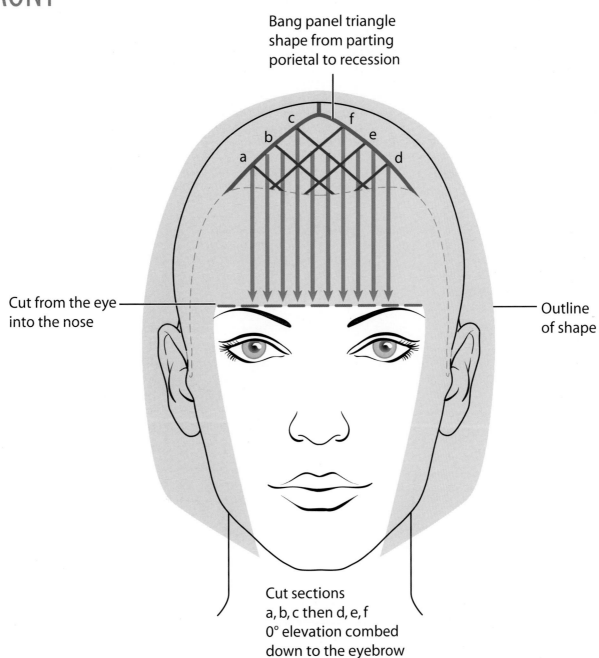

Bang panel triangle shape from parting porietal to recession

Cut from the eye into the nose

Outline of shape

Cut sections a, b, c then d, e, f 0° elevation combed down to the eyebrow

LEFT SIDE

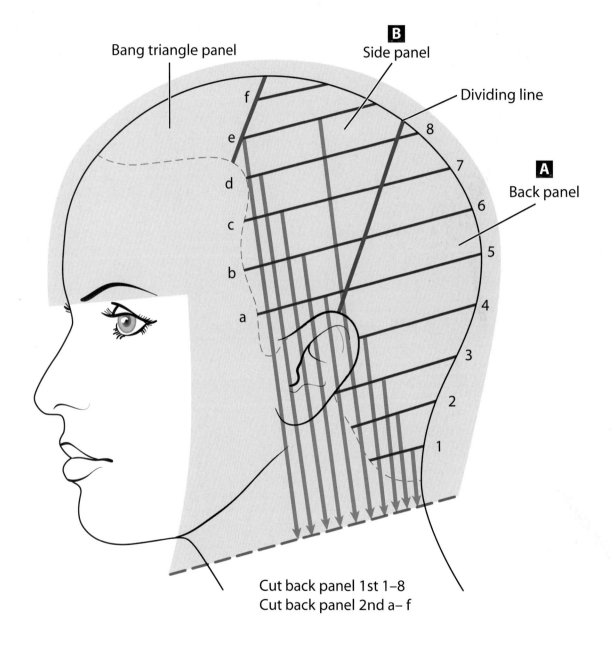

Bang triangle panel

B Side panel

Dividing line

A Back panel

f
e
d
c
b
a

8
7
6
5
4
3
2
1

Cut back panel 1st 1–8
Cut back panel 2nd a– f

RIGHT SIDE

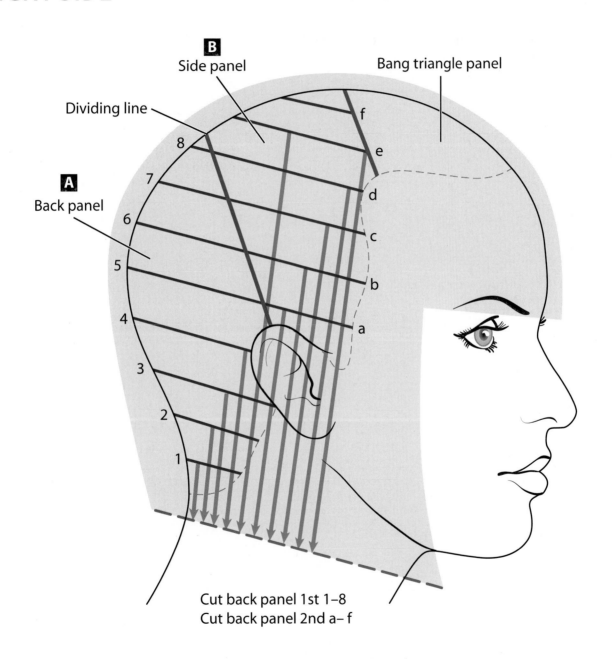

B Side panel

Dividing line

Bang triangle panel

A Back panel

8
7
6
5
4
3
2
1

f
e
d
c
b
a

Cut back panel 1st 1–8
Cut back panel 2nd a– f

BACK

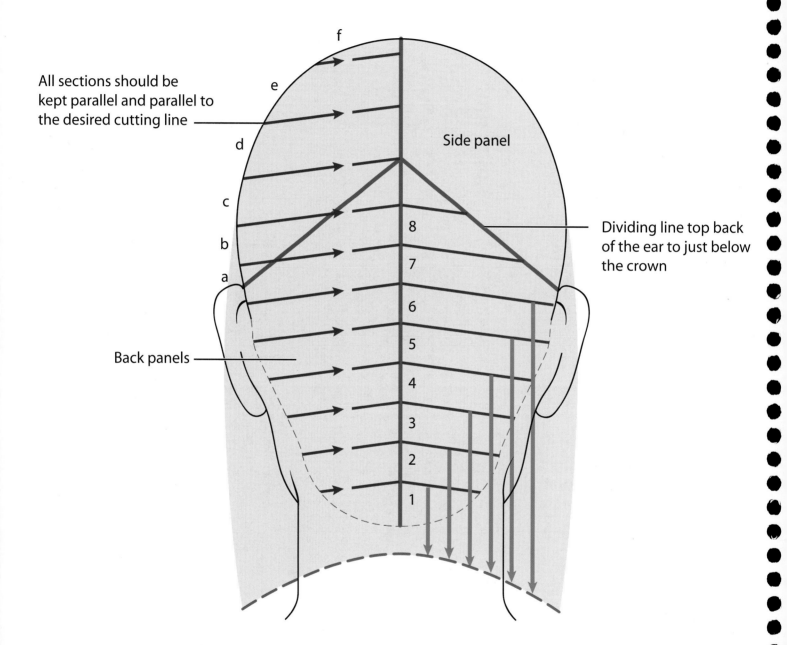

All sections should be kept parallel and parallel to the desired cutting line

Side panel

Dividing line top back of the ear to just below the crown

Back panels

TOP

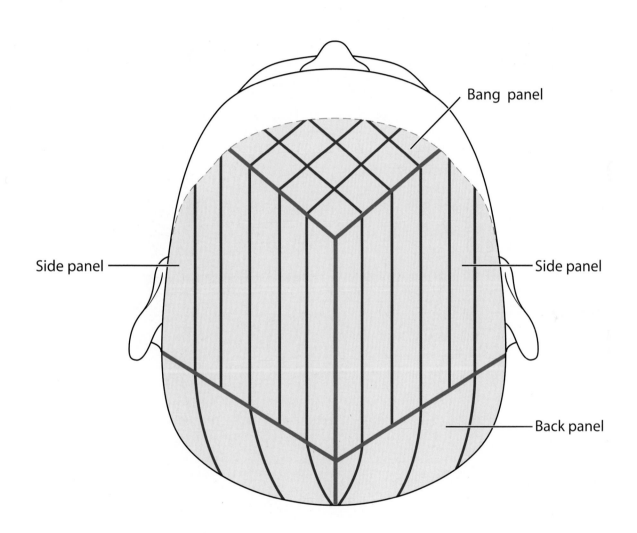

Bang panel

Side panel

Side panel

Back panel

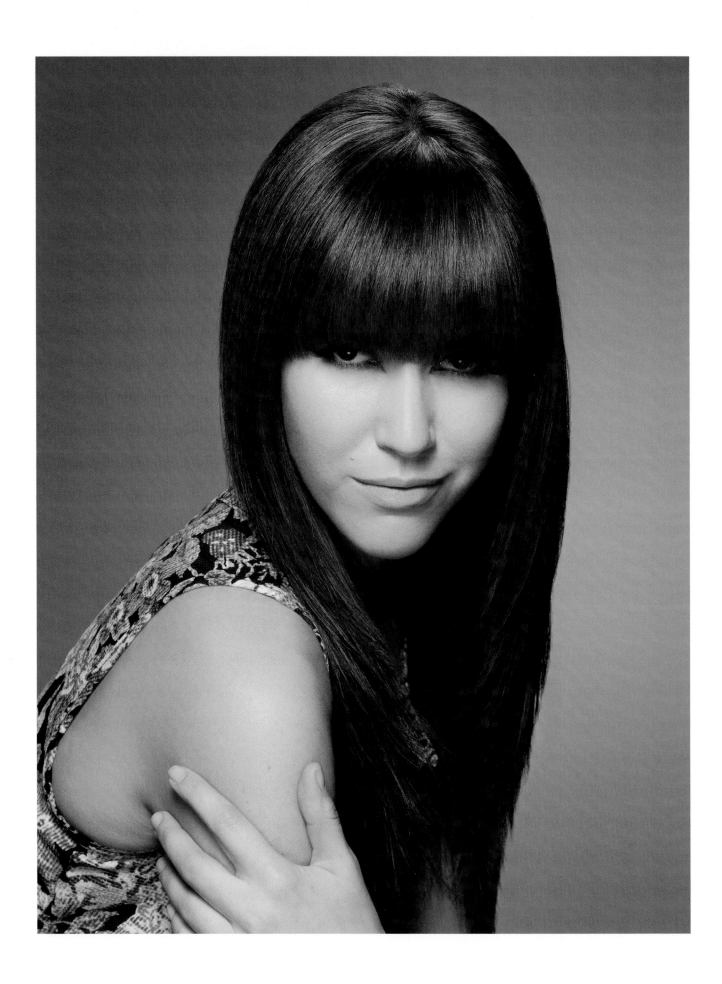

CHAPTER 4

CLASSIC LONG LAYERS

Learning Objectives

After completing this chapter, you will be able to:

☑ LO ❶   Demonstrate the proper positioning to correctly cut the front section of the haircut.

☑ LO ❷   Recognize and identify the correct C-shaped cut from the front hairline to the baseline using the closed blade cutting technique.

☑ LO ❸   Demonstrate how to check for balance both visually and technically.

☑ LO ❹   Implement gradual elevation and overdirection while working from front through to the sides and back.

☑ LO ❺   Execute correct ear-to-ear parting (incorporating the drop back crown) to properly add layers in the back.

☑ LO ❻   Demonstrate how to add light layers to the back of the head while removing the corner weight.

☑ LO ❼   Understand and perform cutting square, choppy bangs using diagonal lines to create texture.

CLASSIC LONG LAYER WITH CHOPPY BANGS

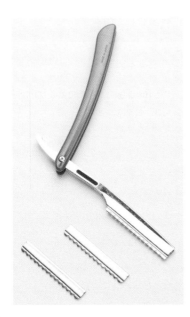

The classic long layer is the type of cut that you can use to build a successful career. It is perhaps the most popular style for a salon client because it is feminine, easy to wear, has some length to it, and adds youthfulness and beauty in a graceful and cultured way. It suits women of any hair type and of any age. If you perfect this cut, you will have many happy clients recommending you to their friends and family. It is a very desirable and client-friendly style. It has the potential to help you build a whole new client base. Executed skillfully, the long layers create an illusion of thickness for finer hair types and conversely, they make thick, coarse hair easier to manage and control, especially as the guarded razor is great for taking out weight. "Long" is defined as hair that falls below the shoulders. The objective of the cut is to create maximum face-framing shape, while retaining the weight and structure of the one-length baseline through the back. There are some key things to keep in mind while practicing this technique. If cutting more than 2 inches (5 cm) of length, you should use the one-length line sectioning pattern (outlined in Chapter 3) and cut the hair to the desired length with no elevation, while holding the hair between your fingers at the appropriate length on the client's back. The sectioning pattern for layers is critical. You must make a deep diagonal parting from the front hairline to the side hairline; this sectioning pattern determines the shape of your face-framing layers. You are using 0-degree elevation at the front (you can build elevation as you move to the back) and you cut in a 'C' shape or curved line from the center and the side, down to the baseline using the closed-blade technique. The balance between the layers on each side is another crucial factor in determining the success of the cut. The choppy bangs add the finishing touch that makes clients go "*Wow!*" Drifting elegantly toward the eyebrows, these wispy, texturized square bangs frame the cheekbones and the eyes, placing the spotlight on women's most beautifying facial features. The cut works with all hair textures, but the natural body and bounce that the style creates seems especially suited to soft and pretty waves. The final style should look and feel lightweight, with lots of freedom and movement.

IMPLEMENTS AND MATERIALS

You will need all of the following implements, materials, and supplies:

- Cutting cape
- Guarded razor
- Neck strip
- Sectioning clips
- Spray bottle with water
- Towels
- Wide-tooth comb
- Blowdryer
- Oval flat brush

PROCEDURE: Classic Long Layer with Choppy Bangs

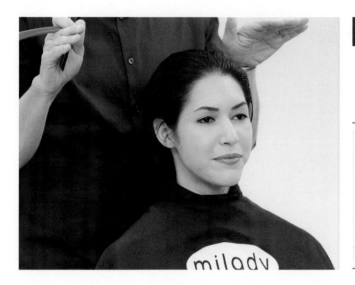

1 Position the client at chest level. The client's head position should be upright, in its natural position, for the entire cut.

HERE'S A **TIP:**

When cutting the long layers in from the front, remember to remain standing in front of the client, moving no further to the side than the arm of the chair. Using the client as a point to pivot from helps to keep layers even and balanced.

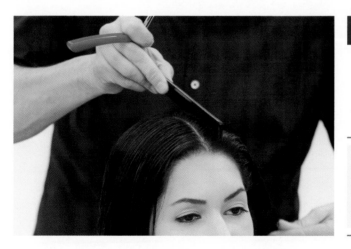

2 Using the wide teeth of the sectioning comb, create a central parting from the front hairline to the top of the head.

HERE'S A **TIP:**

Hairs are combed toward you, always using the fine teeth of the comb for maximum tension.

PROCEDURE: Classic Long Layer with Choppy Bangs

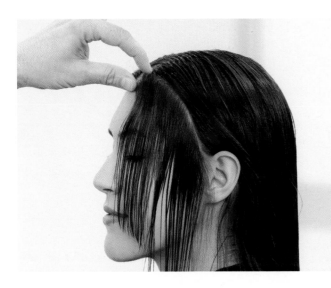

3 Next position yourself directly in front of the client. Begin the cut, starting on your favored side, by creating a half-inch, deep diagonal parting from the front hairline to the side hairline. This section determines the face-framing layers. Comb all hair into natural fall.
☑ LO ❶

HERE'S A **TIP:**

Maintain consistent, even, diagonal sections as you work through the front and sides.

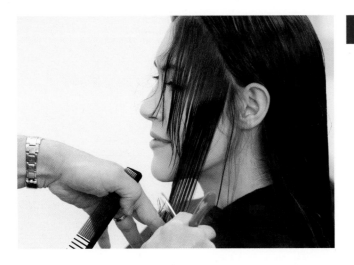

4 Using short cutting strokes with a closed blade, cut in a "C-shape" or curved line from the corner of the mouth down the length with 0-degree elevation and tight tension. The 0-degree, face-framing, "C-shape" angle determines the length and the amount of layering you will create in the front of the face throughout the entire cut. The face frame becomes your guide for your layers throughout the haircut.
☑ LO ❷

PROCEDURE: Classic Long Layer with Choppy Bangs

5 Repeat steps 3 and 4 to create an additional two sections, directly behind the first section on your favored side. ☑ LO❶ ☑ LO❷

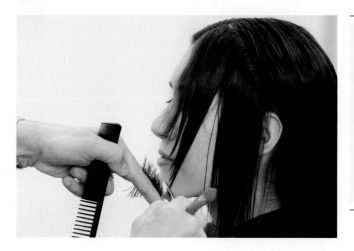

HERE'S A **TIP:**

Although you could cut the whole of one side of your classic long layers and then move to the opposite side, in reality this will make keeping consistent with your guideline very, very difficult because you are gradually building elevation as you work through the sections. So rather than cutting one side and then the other, maintain a back-and-forth practice, going from side to side after every two or three sections.

6 After completing the first three sections on your favored side, move to the opposite side and repeat steps 3 and 4. ☑ LO❶ ☑ LO❷

HERE'S A **TIP:**

There is not a fixed amount of elevation that should be used. The more you elevate, the more you take off; the less you elevate, the longer the hair will be, and the heavier the layer will be. Whether using a little or a lot, the most important thing is to ensure consistent elevation and consistent overdirection throughout the entire haircut.

PROCEDURE: Classic Long Layer with Choppy Bangs

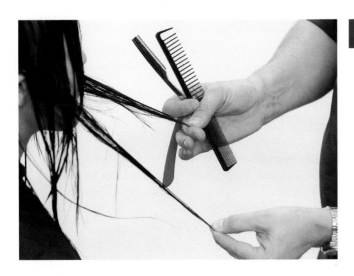

7 Once you have completed the first section on the opposite side, carefully check for balance. Refine as necessary, then repeat steps 4 and 5 to complete the next two sections on this side. ☑ LO❸

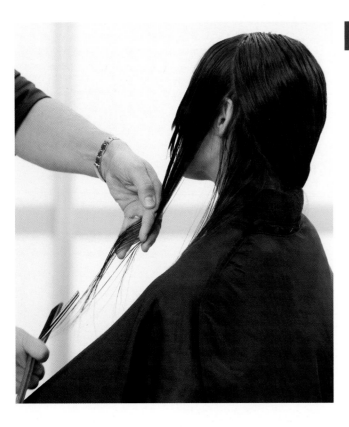

8 Once the face frame has been established on both sides, move back to your favored side. Rotate the head slightly, and create the next diagonal section behind the ear from the top of the head to the nape.

PROCEDURE: Classic Long Layer with Choppy Bangs

9   Slightly overdirect the hair, and with a closed blade, cut with 30-degree elevation as you move down the length. Repeat to create an additional two sections, working toward the back of the head on your favored side. As you progress, the elevation and overdirection continues to build up and out from previously cut sections. ☑ L○④

10   Move to the opposite side, and repeat steps 8 and 9 to create and cut three sections on this side. ☑ L○④

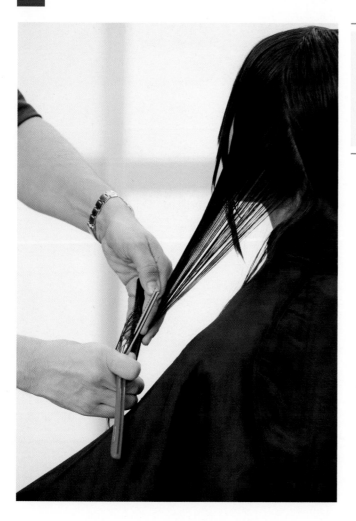

HERE'S A **TIP:**

Keep the client's head still, in the same position, throughout the cut. This enables you to build the shape around the position of the head. This will keep you consistent and make your layering more intricate.

PROCEDURE: Classic Long Layer with Choppy Bangs

11 When you reach the top of the apex, you will start to take sections from this point until reaching the center back. Create the next section from the apex down to the nape, overdirect and cut with gradual elevation and tight tension. Cut an additional two sections, then move and repeat this step on the opposite side. ☑ LO ④

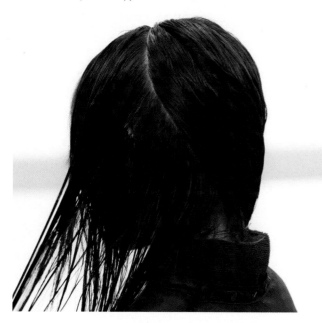
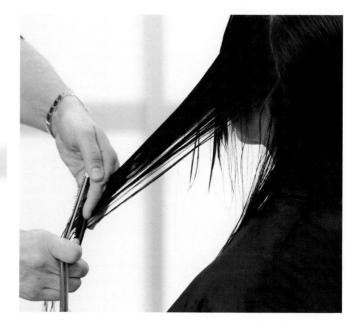

12 Once you have completed both sides, carefully check for balance one last time. Refine as necessary. ☑ LO ③

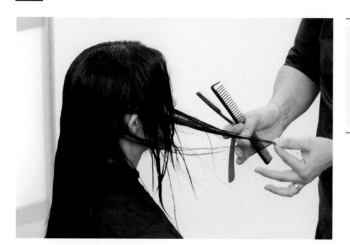

HERE'S A **TIP:**

Remember that this haircut comes down and around. Therefore, you should be making sure that you have created roundness in the shape.

PROCEDURE: Classic Long Layer with Choppy Bangs

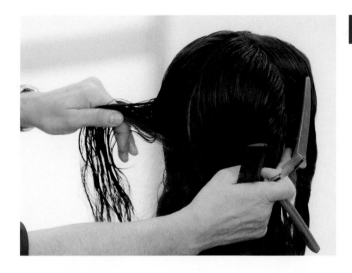

13 To round out the back layers, resection the hair from the top of the head down to the top of each ear.

☑ LO⑤

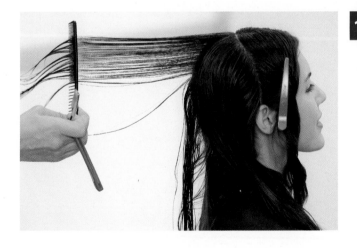

14 Create a 1-inch (2.54-cm) wide section that goes from the center back of the head, down to the nape, using the top of the spine as your guide to keep the section central.

PROCEDURE: Classic Long Layer with Choppy Bangs

15 Using the fine teeth of your comb for maximum tension, comb hair straight out from crown at 90-degree elevation from the head and, while using the closed-blade technique, cut and remove this weight by cutting a curved line to the desired length. This is often referred to as 'removing the corner,' and it is now your guide for the center back layers. ☑ LO❻

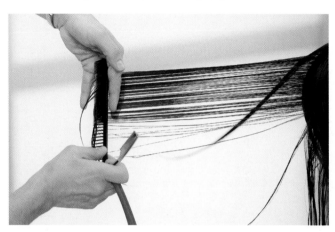 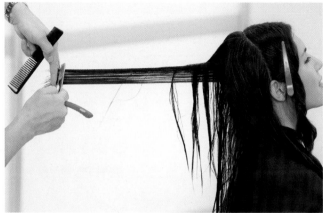

16 When approaching the center back layers, cut your favored side first. Standing on your favored side, take a half-inch vertical section parallel to the guide in the back. Comb hair straight out from the crown and direct back to the center guide; then razor cut hair with a closed blade. Follow the same steps for the opposite side. Do *not* overdirect guide beyond the center; it is vital that your guide remains stationary. ☑ LO❻

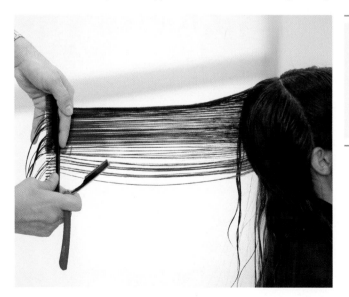

HERE'S A **TIP:**

As there is less layering through the back, you can use the tipping guarded razor technique to add some texture to the back section. This is literally tipping the blade into hair vertically to texturize.

PROCEDURE: Classic Long Layer with Choppy Bangs

17 Complete back layers using the technique outlined in step 16 until you reach the desired length. ☑ LO ⑥

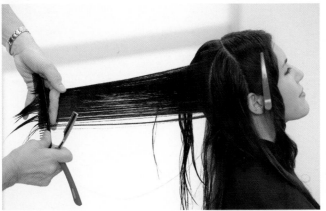

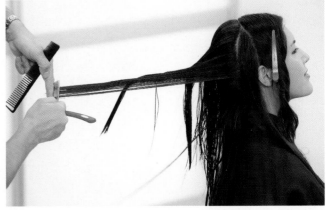

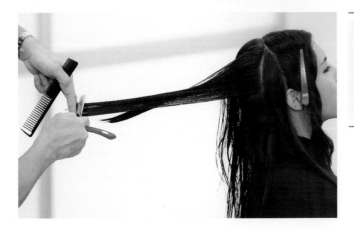

HERE'S A **TIP:**

Check everything visually, as well as technically, as it is the visual aesthetic that keeps hairdressers inspired and clients happy.

PROCEDURE: Classic Long Layer with Choppy Bangs

18 Cross-check layers in the back using the fine teeth of the comb for even, smooth tension and horizontal sections to ensure that there is balance in the layers. Razor cut away any unbalanced pieces, refining the interior shape. ☑ LO❸

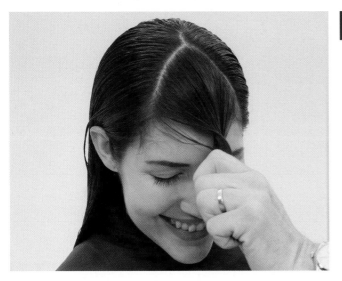

19 Next create the choppy bangs. To begin, make a triangular-shaped section that goes from the parting to the recession. ☑ LO❼

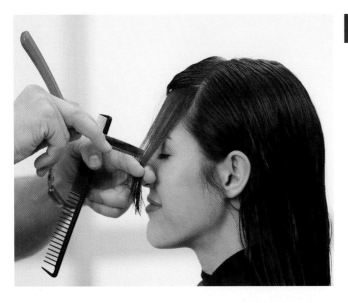

20 Take a 90-degree section from one corner of the triangle. Comb this section straight down, and cut a blunt, straight line to the desired length, usually just above the eyebrow. With wispy bangs, it can be shorter if desired. ☑ LO❼

PROCEDURE: Classic Long Layer with Choppy Bangs

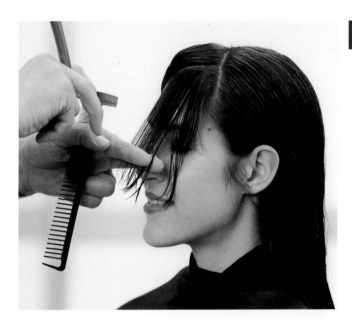

21 From the same side working up the triangle, make and cut two more sections in exactly the same fashion. Comb each section straight down, and cut a blunt, straight line to the desired length. ☑ LO⑦

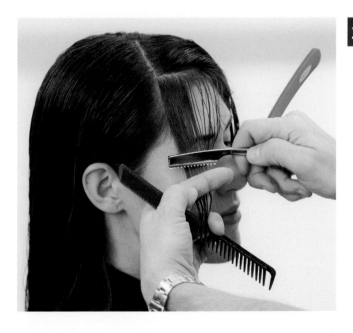

22 Move to the opposite side of your original triangle section, and repeat the process. Once all six sections of the triangle are cut, comb the entire bang section forward to check length and weight.

PROCEDURE: Classic Long Layer with Choppy Bangs

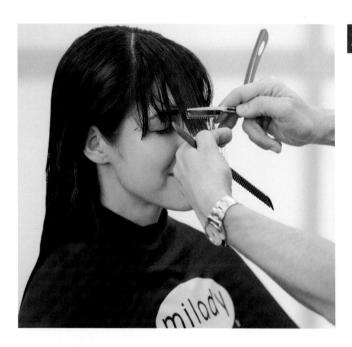

23 Next take the same subsections as before and cut short, slight diagonal lines with even, consistent, comb tension no further than a ½ inch (1.27cm) into the straight line, while using a slightly open blade in order to add more softness and texture. The lines can resemble a zigzag. Release hair and look at the texture created. Remember, this will build as the remaining sections are texturized.

☑ LO ❼

24 If satisfied with the texture, continue onto the remaining subsections of the bangs until reaching the final section. Once complete, comb, check, and refine as necessary.

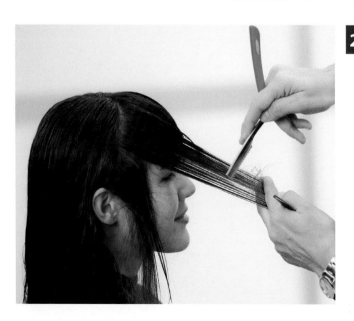

25 To finish the cut, comb out the front layers and cut with a light tipping-out technique using slight elevation and overdirection. Repeat on the opposite side.

☑ LO ❼

PROCEDURE: Classic Long Layer with Choppy Bangs

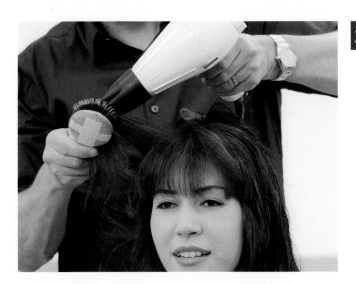

26 Next, using an oval flat brush, blowdry hair smooth so that you can accurately check the quality of the cut. Blowdry the front and sides, and then move to the back, always working from roots to ends.

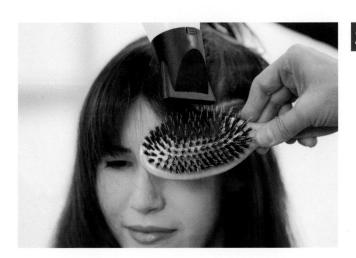

27 For best results, blowdry in sections that reflect the pattern of your cutting sections. Make sure that each section is completely dry before proceeding to the next one.

PROCEDURE: Classic Long Layer with Choppy Bangs

28 With the style complete, layers should fall around the eyes, cheekbones, and chin, drawing attention to features and showing off the perfectly balanced shape of your long layered cut. Check the front and sides in the mirror and from a distance to ensure that each element of the cut—balance, shape, length, and weight—has fallen into place.

HERE'S A **TIP:**

Once you have perfected the technique and are working with clients, you will find different people want different types of blowdry. One client may wish their hair to be smooth and sleek; others may prefer a bend or bevel. You can also blowdry this style wavy or curly. Be sure to choose the right products and brushes, used with the right blowdry techniques, to make your clients happy with the finish.

PERFORMANCE RUBRICS

The following rubrics are used for organizing and interpreting data gathered from observations of performance with regard to this long layered guarded razor haircut. It is a clearly developed scoring document used to differentiate between levels of development in a specific skill or behavior. I recommend they be used as a tool to gauge progress, either through self-assessment or with the aid of your educator. Write down your notes, chart the development of your skills, and vow to never stop learning.

Performance is evaluated according to the following scale:

1. **Development Opportunity:** There is little or no evidence of competency; Assistance is needed; Performance includes multiple errors.

2. **Fundamental:** There is beginning evidence of competency; Task is completed alone; Performance includes few errors.

3. **Competent:** There is detailed and consistent evidence of competency; Task is completed alone; Performance includes rare errors.

4. **Strength:** There is detailed evidence of highly creative, inventive, mature presence of competency. Space is provided for comments to assist you in improving your performance and achieving a higher rating.

Performance Assessed	1	2	3	4	Improvement Plan
Demonstrated correct client body positioning in chair					
Demonstrated correct sectioning patterns for long layers with a guarded razor					
Demonstrated correct 'C'-shaped cutting from front hairline to baseline with 0-degree elevation					
Demonstrated correct amount of hair to cut in each section (half-inch)					
Demonstrated correct and consistent amount of comb tension					
Demonstrated ability to create a strong face frame guideline					
Demonstrated ability to gradually build elevation and overdirection while working from front through to sides and back					
Demonstrated ability to maintain corner length (where face frame meets the baseline)					

Performance Assessed	1	2	3	4	Improvement Plan
Demonstrated ability to cut the apex with 90-degree elevation					
Demonstrated ability to check sections visually, as well as technically, ensuring symmetry and balance					
Demonstrated ability to cross-check through the center, ensuring layers connect from side to side					
Demonstrated correct ear-to-ear parting (incorporating the drop back crown) to razor layers and roundness into the corners in the back					
Demonstrated ability to create right balance of layers, length, and weight					
Demonstrated ability to "tip" out extra weight using the tipping technique with the razor					
Demonstrated ability to cut away any unbalanced pieces, refining the interior shape					
Demonstrated correct sectioning pattern (triangle) for choppy bangs					
Demonstrated correct procedure for razoring bangs in a square line to desired length and then razoring in diagonal lines to create texture					
Demonstrated correct blowdry procedure					
Demonstrated ability to hold the hair in hands correctly in preparation for razoring (see Chapter 2 for thorough explanation of the technique). This should be maintained throughout the entire procedure.					
Demonstrated ability to use a piston-like movement while razoring with a closed blade (see Chapter 2 for thorough explanation of the technique). This should be maintained throughout the entire procedure.					

FRONT

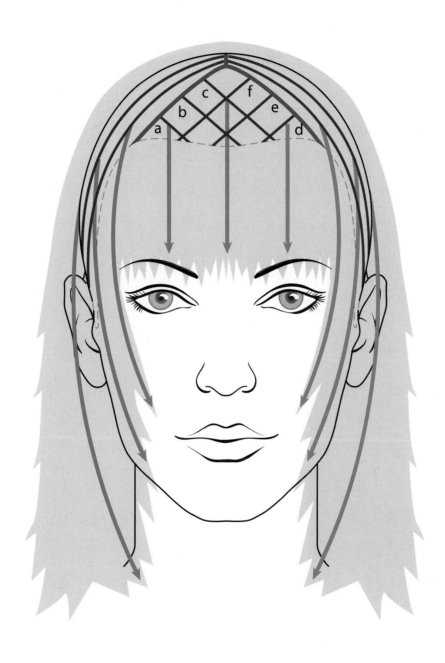

LEFT SIDE

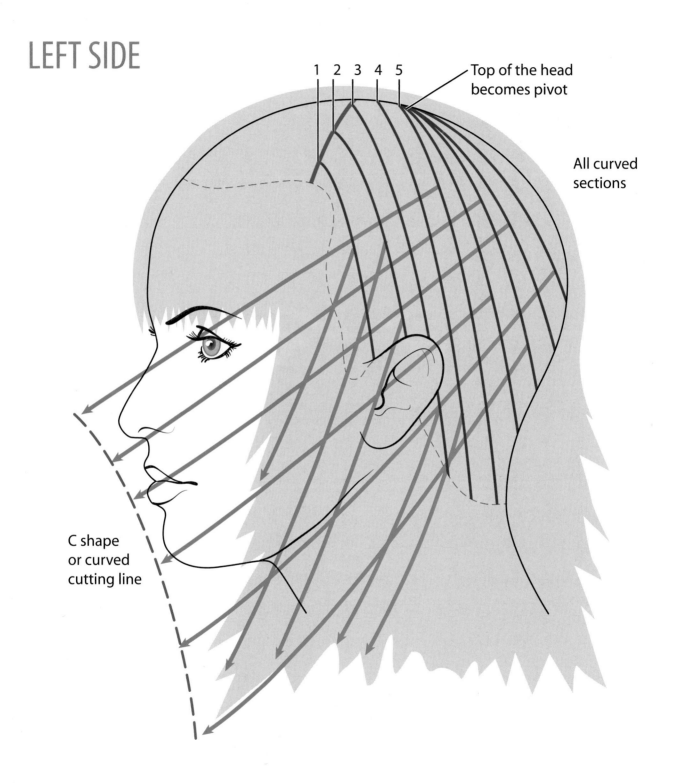

1 2 3 4 5

Top of the head
becomes pivot

All curved
sections

C shape
or curved
cutting line

RIGHT SIDE

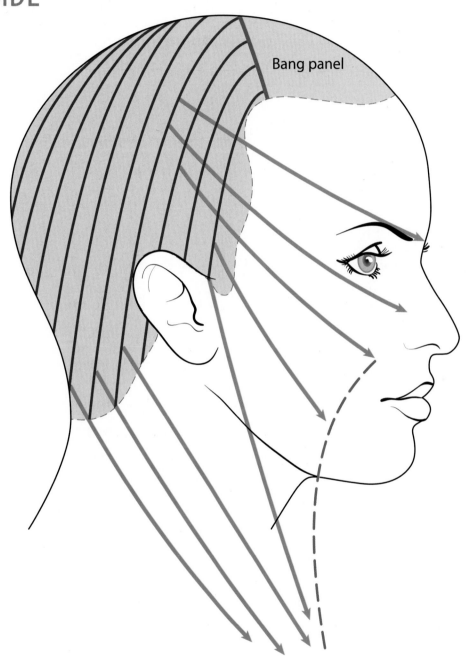

Bang panel

BACK

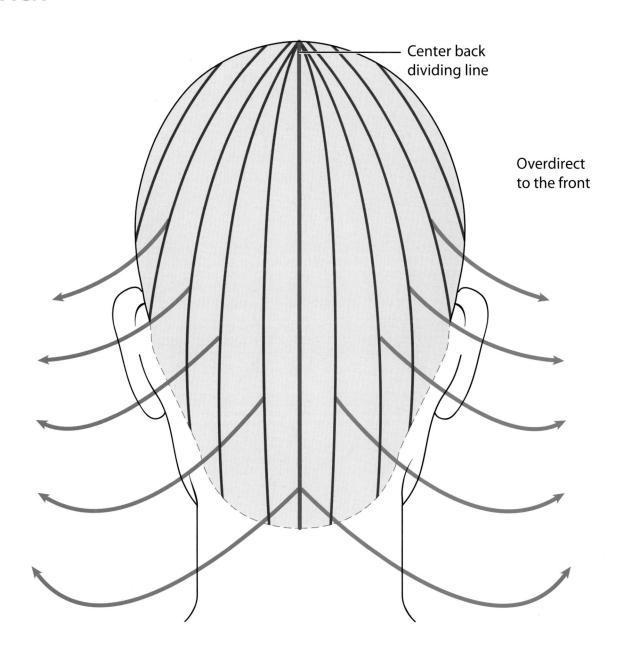

Center back
dividing line

Overdirect
to the front

TOP

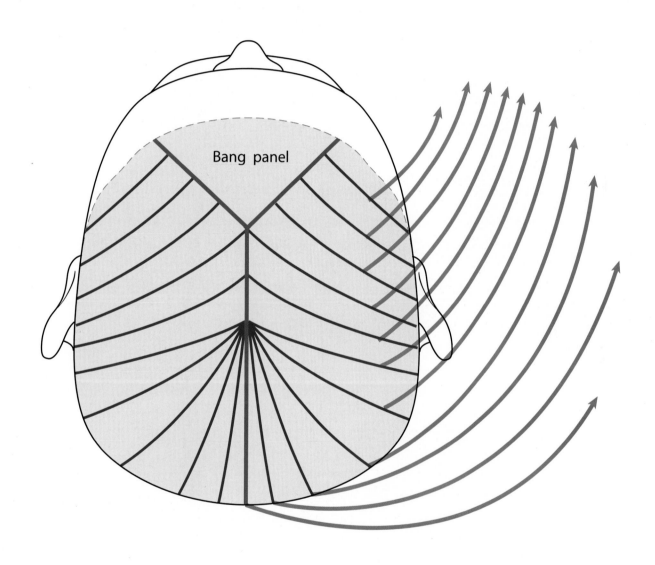

Bang panel

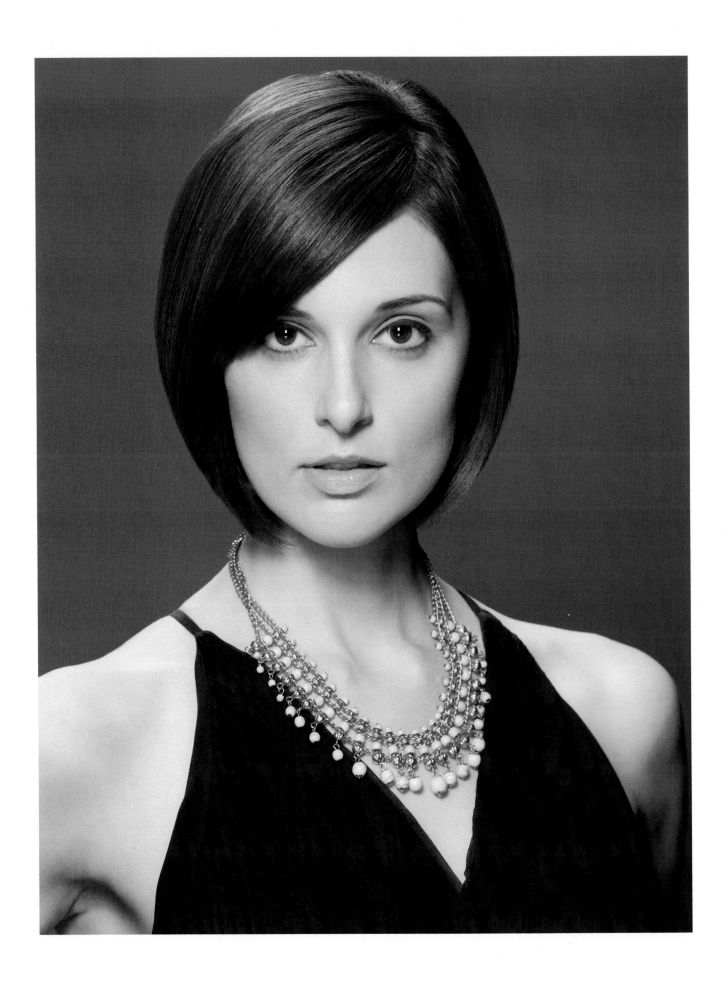

CHAPTER 5
RAZOR GRADUATION

Learning Objectives

After completing this chapter, you will be able to:

☑ ☐ **1** Demonstrate how to create the correct side-part sectioning pattern.

☑ ☐ **2** Demonstrate how to create the first section as a guideline for the rest of the haircut.

☑ ☐ **3** Perform a piston-like razor-cutting motion.

☑ ☐ **4** Implement a steady and consistent open-blade technique to create a graduated shape.

☑ ☐ **5** Demonstrate how to check for balance and how to refine if necessary.

☑ ☐ **6** Demonstrate the open and flat razoring technique to create softness.

☑ ☐ **7** Demonstrate the tipping out razor cutting technique to remove weight.

☑ ☐ **8** Demonstrate how to properly cut both sides of the head, completing the graduated shape of the bob.

BOB WITH GRADUATION AND SIDE-SWEPT BANGS

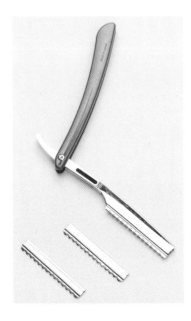

Aesthetically, there are many reasons to love the shape of a bob with graduation, especially when cut with a razor. The graduation through the back helps hair to appear elevated, giving the impression of volume and fullness. The slightly jagged lines of the razor cut aid a feeling of youthful, choppy separation and piece-y-ness. And because this classic and beautifying style is chin length, it creates the perfect frame for features like cheekbones, chin, lips, and eyes—making it the kind of cut that guilds the lily of even the prettiest flower. Less figuratively, it makes clients feel beautiful, young, and refreshed, which means it is a great money-maker in the salon. This cut is the ultimate skill-test, and it is the hardest technical hair cut to execute. Anyone who achieves a perfect razor bob with graduation is considered a master of the razor. The good news is that the sectioning pattern is the same as it is for the one-length guarded razor bob in Chapter 3. The challenge is that the graduation occurs by way of a perfectly timed, steady, and consistent opening and rotating of the blade as you work to take out the right amount of length and density to create a beautifully beveled, graduated shape that sits on the nape with no weight line. This cut is not easy, and it will require that you have complete understanding of the technique, and the visual artistry to know when to "graduate," and by how much. Essentially, when you begin opening the blade, you are taking shorter pieces of hair because your razoring is now going deeper. These shorter pieces on the inside provide even graduation, while the lengths that come to the outline help to create smoothness within a beveled shape. So, remember, the graduation is internal, not external. The cut is a timeless classic, suiting everyone from fashionable girls about town to mature ladies who wear their hair with style and class. It has lots of versatility, too. A smooth blowdry with a few runs of a flatiron will create a sleek, shiny, elongated version; a round brush, curling iron or wand, meanwhile, lets you create lots of full, sexy tousle, with cascading swing and movement. The cut suits all hair types, and it is especially beneficial for thick and coarse hair because of all the weight removal. Perfect this cut and you have proved your craftsmanship and laid the foundations to build your creative stock. Drifting elegantly above the brow, side-swept bangs are great for accenting eyes, and my favorite fringe placement for this cut. Successfully accomplish this soft side swoosh and it is another string to your bow.

IMPLEMENTS AND MATERIAL

You will need all of the following implements, materials, and supplies:

- Cutting cape
- Guarded razor
- Haircutting shears
- Neck strip
- Sectioning clips
- Spray bottle with water
- Towels
- Wide-tooth comb
- Blowdryer
- Flat brush

PROCEDURE: Bob with Graduation and Side-Swept Bangs

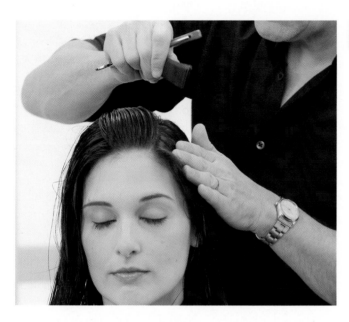

1 Start by creating a side parting by finding the natural separation in the hair. Section the hair from the crown down to the nape, using the top of the spine as your guide for staying central. ☑ LO❶

2 Create the first section on the hairline at the nape. Take a 1/2-inch (1.27-cm), diagonal section from the center parting to the corners of the hairline. ☑ LO❷

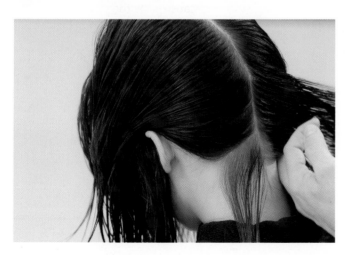 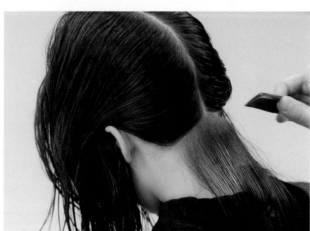

PROCEDURE: Bob with Graduation and Side-Swept Bangs

3 Cut your first section with the closed-blade razor cutting technique to establish the guideline from the center of the nape toward the back of the ear. The first section is always the most important because it is your guide for the rest of the cut; with that in mind, focus on cutting this section with maximum precision. Always work from the center nape to the back of each ear; naturally, on one side you will cut with the heel of the razor, on the other you will cut with the tip of the razor. ☑ LO❷

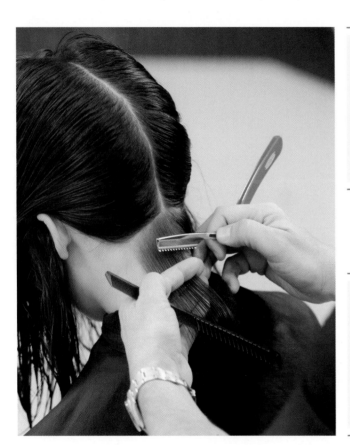

HERE'S A **TIP:**

Work with the wide teeth of the comb to comb the hair around as you check sections, balance, length and weight. Work with the narrow teeth of the comb as you prepare each section for the cut. The narrow teeth are better for maintaining good tension; the wide teeth are better for combing hair around freely and easily.

HERE'S A **TIP:**

Remember that you are cutting across the hairline at the back of the neck; a square line at the nape will, therefore, have the appearance of a very slight arch, just as the neck does. Because of this, your sections should be on a slight diagonal—not quite horizontal, not quite diagonal, but in between, so that it mimics your cutting line on the nape.

PROCEDURE: Bob with Graduation and Side-Swept Bangs

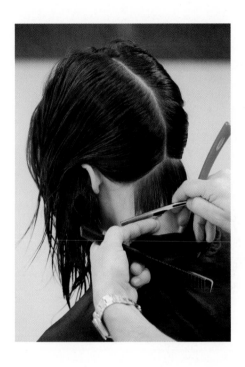

4 Continue up the head in parallel subsections, always working from the center out using the closed-blade technique, a methodical, piston-like motion, and 0-degree elevation.
☑ LO ❸

HERE'S A **TIP:**

With your comb, make sections of hair that are fine enough so that you can clearly see your guide, and thick enough to cut the hair relatively quickly, while maintaining a good strong tension that you can feel to be taut. Typically, picking up sections of hair that are about a 1/2-inch (1.3-cm) thick is perfect.

5 As you prepare each section for the cut, comb hair straight down from roots to ends. There should be 0-degree elevation at the baseline and even, consistent tension throughout. Once the section is prepared, hold that section of hair between the index finger and middle finger (as outlined in the How to Hold Hair for the Perfect Razor Cut section of Chapter 2) and make your cut.

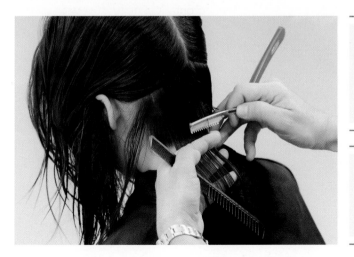

HERE'S A **TIP:**

Maintain fluid, even strokes for consistent graduation. The razor should move like a piston, and the motion should start before you reach the hair.

HERE'S A **TIP:**

If you complete one side before starting the other, maintaining consistency is harder.

PROCEDURE: Bob with Graduation and Side-Swept Bangs

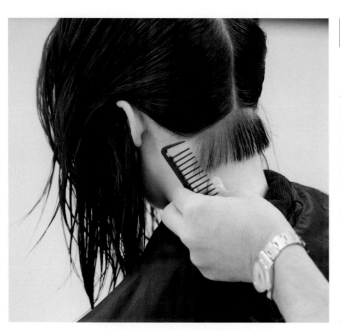

6 Once you have built the outline using the closed blade for a clean, consistent baseline, it is time to start using a more open blade to create the graduated effect with the razor.
☑ LO ④

HERE'S A **TIP:**

The first graduated section is the third section that you will take. When you reach this point, open the blade by about half an inch (1.3 cm), rotate the blade, and use open strokes to cut deep into the interior of the hair. Remember that the piston-like movement of the razor (outlined in the Moving and Rotating the Razor section of Chapter 2) is the key to the success of any razor cut. If the open-blade technique is practiced correctly, you will immediately begin to see more texture as all the hair is no longer falling to the exterior line.

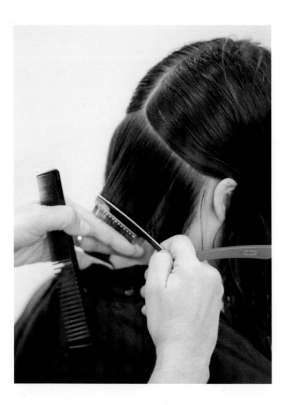

7 Once you get to section 4, open and rotate the blade and slightly elevate as you cut through the section.
☑ LO ④

HERE'S A **TIP:**

Because you are changing density as well as weight, the razor cut bob with graduation gives you a great opportunity to get engaged with the hair. Comb it around as you cut, *feeling* the amount of weight you have taken out.

PROCEDURE: Bob with Graduation and Side-Swept Bangs

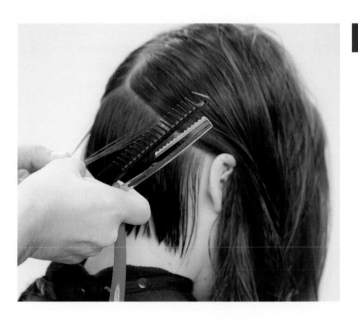

8 Repeat step 7 as you work up the back of the head. Once you get to the occipital bone, check for weight and balance. Refine as necessary.
☑ LO❹

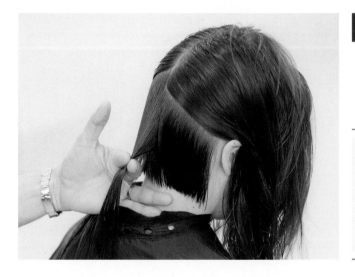

9 Keep checking the consistency of your sections. Sections should be fine enough to see the guide, yet thick enough to take enough hair out and create enough tension.
☑ LO❺

HERE'S A **TIP:**

Keep hair evenly saturated as you razor cut. If hair is too dry, you can shatter the tips too much; too wet, and you will not be able to see the character of the hair texture take shape.

PROCEDURE: Bob with Graduation and Side-Swept Bangs

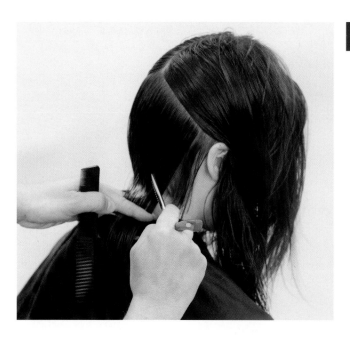

10 Continue working in parallel sections to the section below the crown, to the back of the ear. Gradually increase elevation as you open the blade to create more texture and taper.
☑ LO ❹

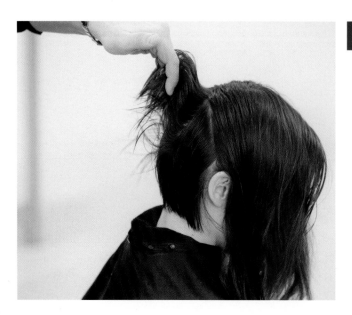

11 Remember that you are removing density as well as length, so make sure you are checking the length and weight of the graduation visually as well as technically. To check, put fingers in hair and pull toward you to feel the thickness and the length.
☑ LO ❺

PROCEDURE: Bob with Graduation and Side-Swept Bangs

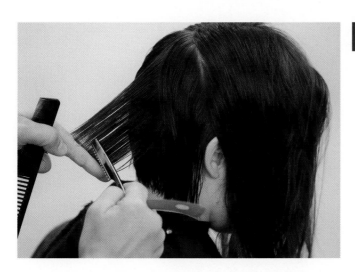

12 If you need to remove more density, you can use the very edge of the blade to "tip out" the density, creating more texture. When cut correctly, the graduation will bevel in toward the head; if the bevel is inconsistent or too thick, it is your sign to tip out more weight. ☑ LO❼

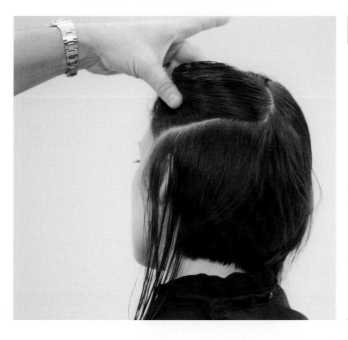

13 Once you reach the horizontal ear-to-ear section, you have completed the back and it is time to move to the sides. As you prepare to work up to the side parting, position the client's head upright and slightly tilted away from you. ☑ LO❽

HERE'S A **TIP:**

Do not worry about unruly bits or an inconsistent hairline. Any problem areas can be cleaned up at the end; first focus on maintaining proper technique as you graduate the shape.

PROCEDURE: Bob with Graduation and Side-Swept Bangs

14 The hair in the section behind the ear can be combed back and razored using the previously cut guideline from the back. Be sure to maintain the length of the exterior line, while creating shorter, textured pieces on the interior; this is vital for achieving a balanced graduation. ☑ LO ❽

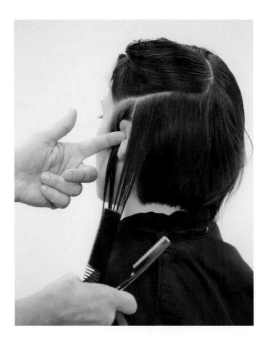

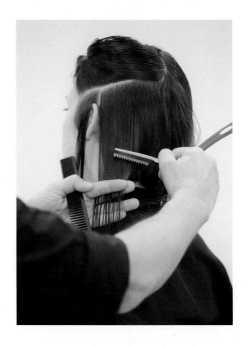

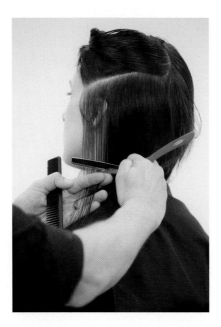

15 For the hair in the section in front of the ear, ignore the ear and comb straight over it, making a section that is bigger than usual to ensure this section creates a strong guide for the rest of the side. Keep the razor closed to create a clean outline, as in the back. ☑ LO ❽

HERE'S A **TIP:**

Though you should take as much time as you need to become familiar with the cut, once you are practiced and more confident, try to work relatively quickly. Because you are relying on your ability to open and rotate the blade at a consistent angle, working quickly helps you remember how much you have opened the blade. If you take too long between the sections, it is easy to forget just how much graduation you have put in.

PROCEDURE: Bob with Graduation and Side-Swept Bangs

16 When combing and preparing to cut the sides, always overdirect slightly back to maintain length in the front. ☑ LO❽

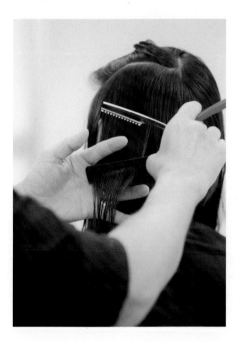

17 As you move up toward the parting, use elevation and an open blade to make the deeper interior cuts that will create graduation through the side. Close the blade as you work down to the ends, ensuring you maintain the outline.
☑ LO❹
☑ LO❽

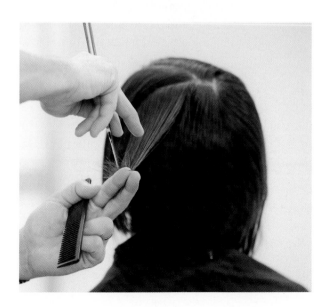

18 Before moving to the opposite side, comb hair out at 90-degrees, overdirecting back as you eliminate bulk by tipping out the weight.
☑ LO❽

PROCEDURE: Bob with Graduation and Side-Swept Bangs

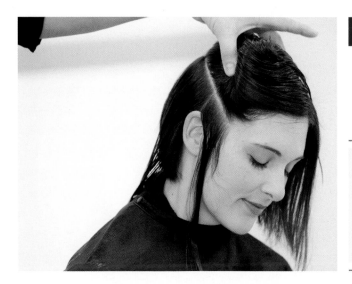

19 Cut your remaining side by repeating steps 13-18. Be sure your client's head is upright and tilted slightly away from you.
☑ LO **8**

HERE'S A **TIP:**

You are working to create a clean exterior with a texturized interior. This allows the hair to bevel in at the back, creating a beautiful, curved shape. There should be no weight on the baseline at the back.

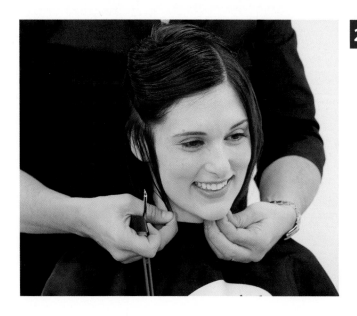

20 Remember to cross-check sections on both sides for balance. This is done by sectioning evenly on both sides and cross-checking your line on every new section. You should also use a mirror to visually check the line; a mirror enables a side-by-side comparison.
☑ LO **5**

PROCEDURE: Bob with Graduation and Side-Swept Bangs

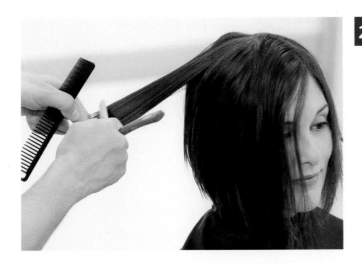

21 As you get to the top of the head, razor the top pieces in small sections in exactly the same fashion as before—opening the blade on the interior to create texture and graduation, while closing the blade toward the ends to maintain the outline. If you feel the top surface is getting too weak, use the open blade a little less—you can always use the tipping technique to remove extra density once the shape is complete.
☑ LO ❻

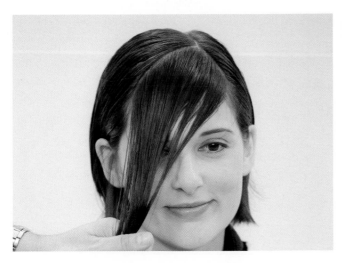

22 To section for side-swept bangs, create a triangle-shaped section from the parting to the recession.

HERE'S A **TIP:**

Because of the combination of technique and feel, and the need to use techniques like overdirection and an open blade, the bob with graduation provides a great technical foundation for all kinds of hairdressing. Learn, practice, and master the technique, and you can use this knowledge to build your creative repertoire.

PROCEDURE: Bob with Graduation and Side-Swept Bangs

23 Taking subsections at 90 degrees, or T to the part, cut at a downward angle toward the lip with the heel of the blade. Cut hair short to long until desired length is reached. Comb hair forward to ensure you have obtained the desired length. The desired length is now your guide for cutting the remaining bang sections.

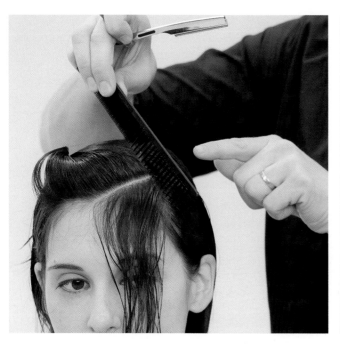

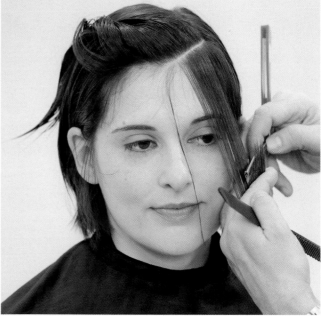

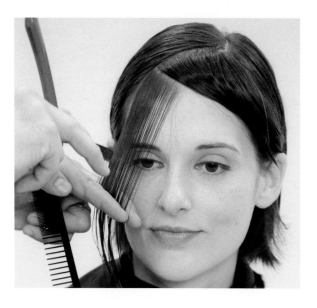

24 On the opposite side, repeat step 23 to make and cut three sections on each side of the face, creating a sweeping V-shaped bang. As you cut each side of the bangs, be mindful to keep the blade away from the client's face. To do so, cut with the heel or the tip of the blade as appropriate, always keeping the body of the blade as far from the face as possible.

PROCEDURE: Bob with Graduation and Side-Swept Bangs

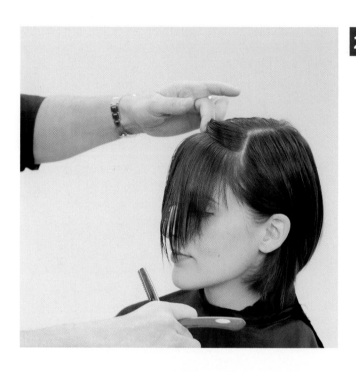

25 Continue taking diagonal sections, and cut to the guide until both sides are complete. Comb hair forward to ensure desired length and weight has been met.

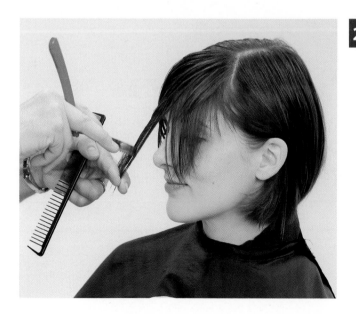

26 Lighten the bangs by taking a 1-inch (2.5-cm) section underneath the top section, and use the tipping technique to take out the excess hair. The idea is to lighten the underneath while maintaining length along the top surface.

PROCEDURE: Bob with Graduation and Side-Swept Bangs

27 Check and refine as needed with shears. LO ⑤

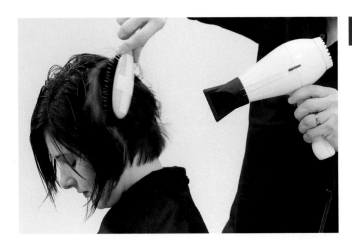

28 Once the cut is complete, blowdry the style straight. Using a flat brush, dry from roots to ends taking 1-inch (2.5-cm) sections, working up the head in sections that mimic your cutting lines. Blowdry with only a little root lift, making sure the amount of root lift is consistent throughout. The integrity of the finish can be compromised if this is not achieved, which makes it more difficult to accurately check your graduation.

PERFORMANCE RUBRICS

The following rubrics are used for organizing and interpreting data gathered from observations of performance regarding this razor cut bob with graduation. It is a clearly developed scoring document used to differentiate between levels of development in a specific skill or behavior. I recommend they be used as a tool to gauge progress, either through self-assessment or with the aid of your educator. Write down your notes, chart the development of your skills, and vow to never stop learning.

Performance is evaluated according to the following scale:

1. **Development Opportunity:** There is little or no evidence of competency; Assistance is needed; Performance includes multiple errors.

2. **Fundamental:** There is beginning evidence of competency; Task is completed alone; Performance includes few errors.

3. **Competent:** There is detailed and consistent evidence of competency; Task is completed alone; Performance includes rare errors.

4. **Strength:** There is detailed evidence of highly creative, inventive, mature presence of competency. Space is provided for comments to assist you in improving your performance and achieving a higher rating.

Performance Assessed	1	2	3	4	Improvement Plan
Demonstrated correct client body positioning in chair					
Demonstrated correct sectioning technique in the back sections					
Demonstrated correct amount of hair to cut in each section (half-inch[1.27cm])					
Demonstrated correct amount of comb tension					
Demonstrated 0-degree elevation while combing hair in preparation for the cutting of the first sections in the back					
Demonstrated ability to cut to desired length in a square line using closed razor blade technique					
Demonstrated ability to maintain fluid, even strokes with the razor					

Performance Assessed	1	2	3	4	Improvement Plan
Demonstrated ability to use first section as guide for the rest of the cut					
Demonstrated ability to begin graduating the cut at the right time, using the open-blade technique					
Demonstrated ability to razor shorter pieces on the interior, yet maintain the exterior line					
Demonstrated ability to continue to build graduation by elevating with comb while overdirecting backward to maintain length					
Demonstrated ability to check sections visually as well as technically					
Demonstrated ability to remove unwanted density by using the tipping technique					
Demonstrated ability to accurately resection side sections in preparation for razoring					
Demonstrated ability to overdirect back, to maintain length in the front, while combing the sides in preparation to cut					
Demonstrated ability to gradually build graduation through the sides, opening the blade while working up toward the parting, and closing the blade on the ends to maintain the outline					
Demonstrated ability to cross-check the two side sections for balance					
Demonstrated ability to judge where the top pieces of hair should fall, while creating graduation on the interior and maintaining length on the outline					
Demonstrated ability to create correct triangle section for side-swept bangs					

Performance Assessed	1	2	3	4	Improvement Plan
Demonstrated ability to cut side-swept bangs to desired length using diagonal sections					
Demonstrated correct blowdry procedure					
Demonstrated ability to properly check and, if necessary, refine finished bob with graduation					
Demonstrated ability to hold the hair in hands correctly in preparation for razoring (see Chapter 2 for thorough explanation of the technique). This should be maintained throughout the procedure.					
Demonstrated ability to use a piston-like movement while razoring with a closed blade and an open blade (see Chapter 2 for thorough explanation of the technique). This should be maintained throughout the procedure.					

FRONT

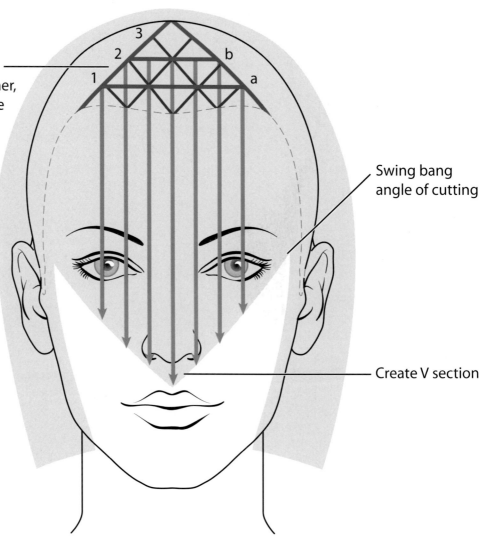

Once the shape of the bangs has come together, in sections a & b use the tipping technique to lighten and soften the bangs from the underneath, while also maintaining length.

Swing bang angle of cutting

Create V section

LEFT SIDE

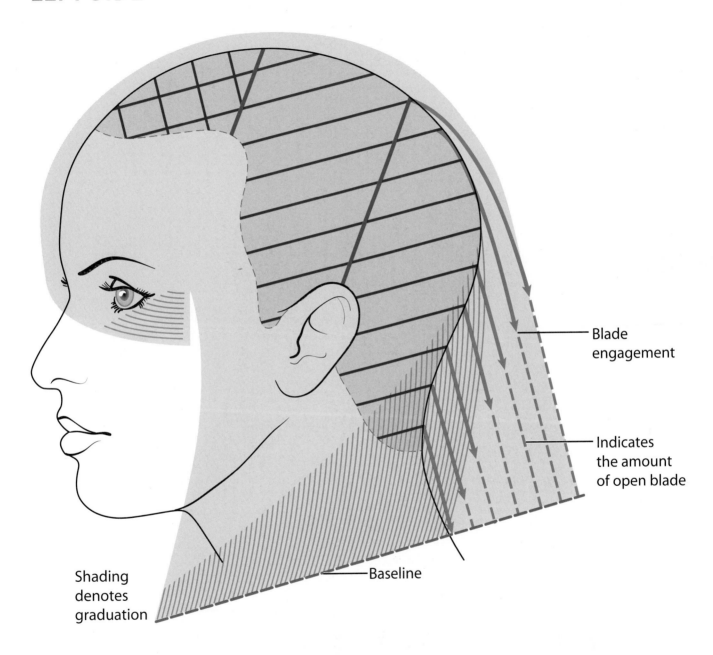

Blade
engagement

Indicates
the amount
of open blade

Shading
denotes
graduation

Baseline

HEADSHEETS

RIGHT SIDE

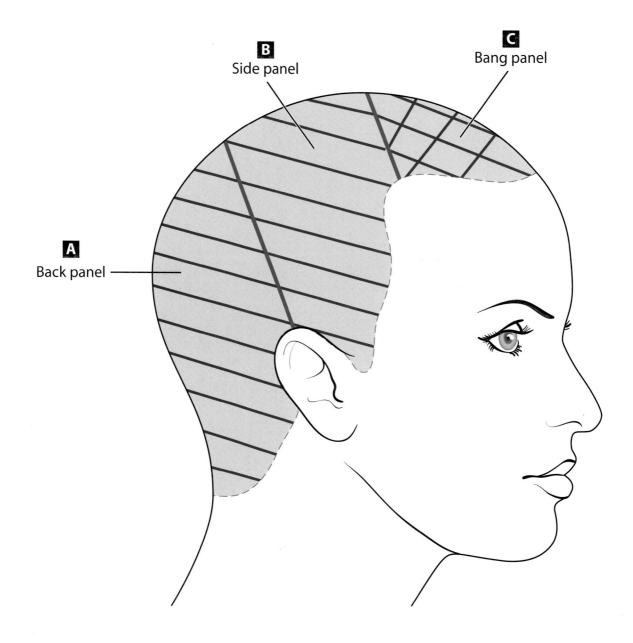

B Side panel

C Bang panel

A Back panel

BACK

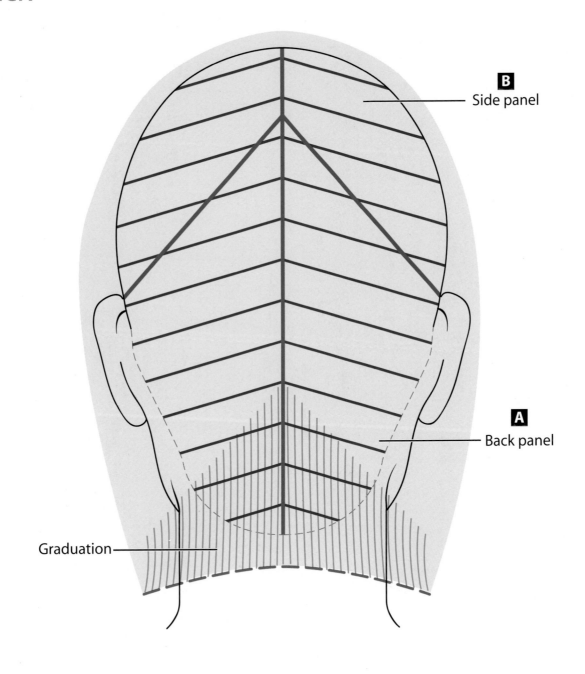

B — Side panel

A — Back panel

Graduation —

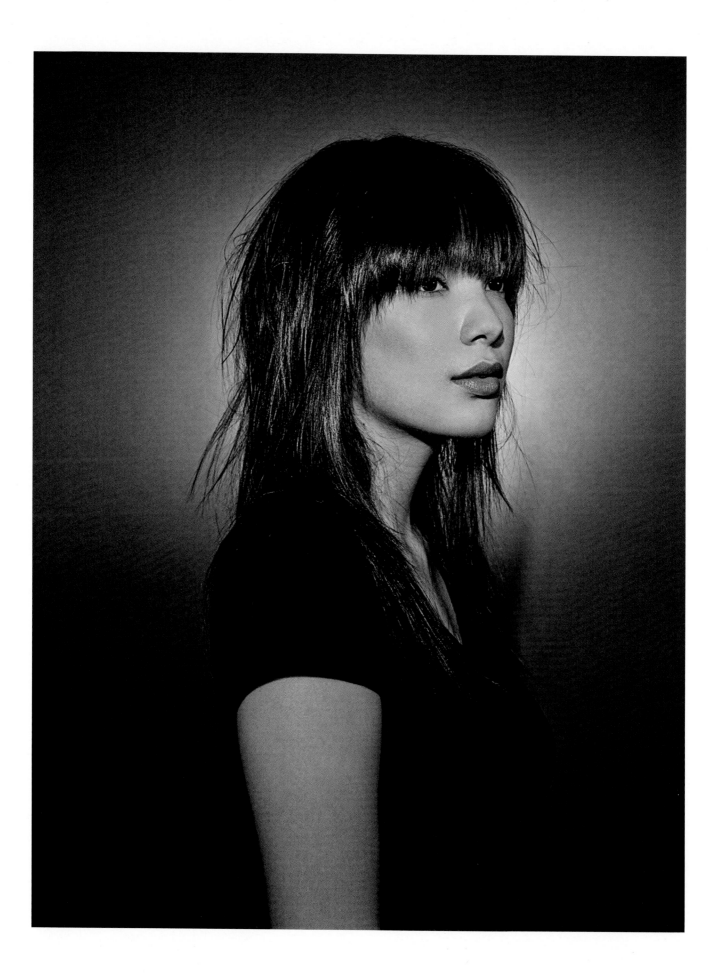

CHAPTER 6

THE RAZOR AND YOU

Learning Objectives

After completing this chapter, you will be able to:

☑ LO ❶ Articulate a basic understanding of the New Shag haircut; specifically, how using asymmetry and disconnection can be used for creative razor cutting.

☑ LO ❷ Describe a *Tri-Plex* haircut and which hair textures it is ideal for.

☑ LO ❸ List three ways you can stay fresh with up-to-date techniques.

☑ LO ❹ Name at least three contemporary razor cuts.

☑ LO ❺ Name a variety of ways the razor can be used for short, mid-length, and long hair styles.

☑ LO ❻ Identify and describe the various career pathways available to stylists.

PAYING IT FORWARD: AFTER THE FUNDAMENTALS

The procedures discussed in Chapters 3 through 5 are the fundamentals of cutting lines, layers, and graduations with your razor. You will need to practice them for thousands of hours to become proficient. When you do master these fundamentals, you enter a world of creative freedom and career opportunities (Figure 6-1). As a beginner stylist, it is exciting and inspiring to think about where this journey may take you. There is so much more to learn about cutting hair with a razor, especially when you are experienced enough to take off the guard and use the unguarded razor. And despite much of the industry's reluctance to switch to razor cutting, razored hairstyles are now so prevalent at the forefront of fashion and beauty trends that being one of its champions gives you a jump on the competition. As such in this final chapter, the idea is to offer a taste of some advanced razoring techniques so you can see the potential to take the skill to the next level. You will examine modern razor cuts, seeing how these styles are tailored to clients in the real world. Finally, I will give you some thoughts on making your way in the industry.

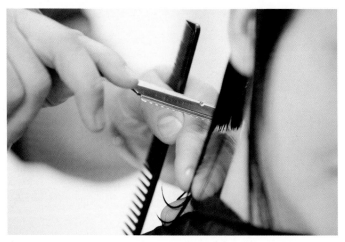

▲ Figure 6-1 The razor is an extension of your mind's eye; the creative cutting possibilities are extraordinary.

CREATIVE POTENTIAL

Creatively, once you master the fundamentals, you can experiment with different techniques, while having your foundations to fall back on. Rather than only cutting layers, lines, and graduations, you can work on asymmetrical shapes, deconstructed lines, graphic undercuts, and lots of other good stuff.

LO ❶ **Articulate a basic understanding of the New Shag haircut; specifically, how using asymmetry and disconnection can be used for creative razor cutting.**

A few years ago, I created a haircut called *The New Shag* (Figure 6-2). Technically, this long hairstyle uses soft asymmetry to bring balance to a unique shape—one that is round on one side, square on the other. The square

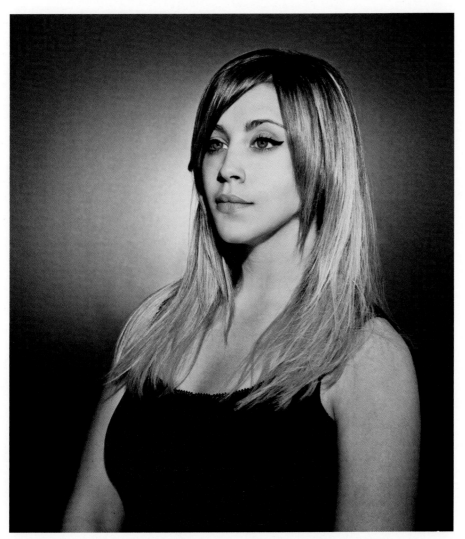

▲ **Figure 6-2** The "New Shag" uses advanced techniques like disconnection and asymmetry.

side is kept flat with super-short undercutting on a horizontal plane. This creates a disconnection that allows another section of (long) hair to fall over the top of the undercut portion, keeping that side of the style light and loose and long and flat. Conversely, the other side is heavier, textured, and *rounded*. To create this rounded shape, I invented a triangular sectioning pattern, which is cut using an experimental, spiraling, windmill-shaped layering technique. The result is a fashionable haircut with space, multitexture, and versatility. The different lengths of hair hit different spots for a soft and shimmering look. Longer lengths and disconnections blend for movement and flexibility within perfect face-framing shape. The style encourages fullness and body and, because of the internal structure of the shape, it can be styled wavy, curly, or straight. With one side shaggy, loose, and round, and the other side slim-lined, sleek, and square, there is a smooth and graceful, visually interesting transition of texture. It is also easy to tailor to different lengths, so I can take it shorter or longer as preference dictates. As a sign of what this kind of invention can do for your career, this look has been featured in fashion, beauty, and trade magazines and websites, and at international beauty shows.

LO ❷ **Describe a *Tri-Plex* haircut and which hair textures it is ideal for.**

This is only one of many examples. More recently, my team and I worked on a cut called *Tri-Plex* (**Figure 6-3**). The idea was to create a new mid-length razor cut for textured hair. Using internal disconnection, external, short to long layering, and a sharp fringe to create three levels within the shape, we invented a progressive, deliberately lived-in look with elegant flowing movement. It is great for wavy-and-curly-haired clients who want to embrace their texture and stay trendy.

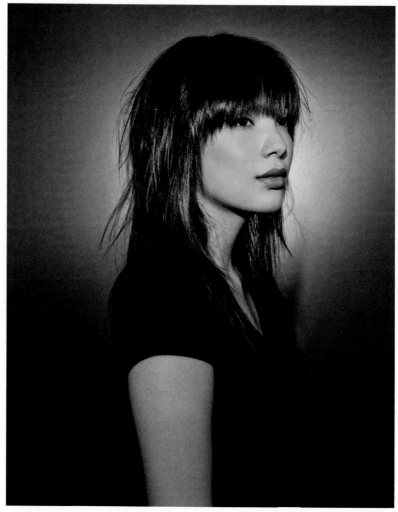

▲ **Figure 6-3** The "Tri-Plex" razor cut was invented with young, fashionable clients in mind.

LO ❸ **List three ways you can stay fresh with up-to-date techniques.**

I hope this helps you to see the potential of this tool to have a positive effect on your craft and career. If you are inspired to continue to improve your razor cutting, search out advanced education from experienced razor cutters. I recommend that you attend hair and beauty shows and educational seminars because it is important to stay fresh, inspired, and aware of what is happening around you. It is also the perfect chance to pick up new ideas which can add to

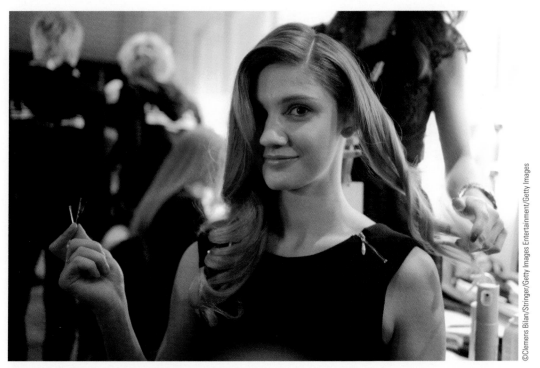

▲ **Figure 6-4** As a master of the craft, the future is yours.

your own repertoire. I would love to see the next generation of original razor cuts coming from you. Learn, practice, master, and the cuts of the future are in your mind's eye (**Figure 6-4**).

CONTEMPORARY RAZOR CUTS

Theory, technique, and practice are all essential, but how do razor cuts work in the real world? It is time now to take a look at how real razor cuts work for real women. Each of the following styles is a modern classic and highlights the youthful and contemporary looks you can create for your clients. More importantly, all these cuts are easy to manage, care for, and style at home. This is another vital ingredient of the successful hairdresser: You must be able to give your clients styles that they can style easily themselves. Clients want to wear great hair every day, not just the day of their salon visit. And this is good for you, too. Your client is your best advertisement. If they have the great hair strut, people will ask, *"Where did you get your hair cut?"* That could and should be you!

LO ❹ Name at least three contemporary razor cuts.

Hip Short Styles

The Choppy Bob and Bangs

This is a youthful, choppy bob with bangs. Through the back, it has been razor cut to the nape to build structure and allow the hair to become elevated, which adds an impression of volume. The razor was used to put in some random layers and take out weight from the interior, giving the style the separation and piece-y-ness that shatters the shape, yet in a soft, structured, and beautiful way. There is no definitive line in the bangs. They were razored to be texturized, moveable, carefree, and easy, while showcasing the model's eyes. A great cut for a hip, young girl because it is modern and cool, yet an easy and fun way to wear the hair (**Figure 6-5**).

The Whimsical Pixie

This short, choppy, and whimsical pixie cut has a few longer, wispy pieces through the back, as opposed to a typical pixie cut, which is kept short all around. For this model, it helped to retain a touch more femininity (**Figure 6-6**). This is a good example of adapting creatively to your client. At first, the cut started out as a classic pixie, but by keeping a bit of extra length in the back, the cut was modified and tailored to help the look remain delicate and graceful. Overall, the style brings out the features in the model's face, while the choppy bangs drift elegantly toward the eyes.

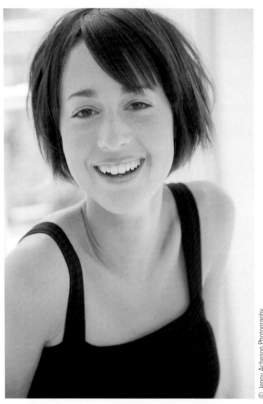

▲ **Figure 6-5** Create youthfulness and beauty, and your clients will always be happy.

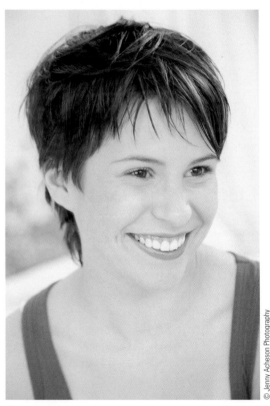

▲ **Figure 6-6** Fuss-free yet beautifying hairstyles will always be popular.

LO ❺ Name a variety of ways the razor can be used for short, mid-length, and long hair styles.

Rounded Razor Graduation with Sweeping Bangs

This model's hair is lovely and thick, so she was a great candidate for a super-chic look, and one that also helps her dense tresses become easier to manage (**Figure 6-7**). A short, razor graduation with sweeping bangs swooshing across the eye line, it has been heavily layered all through the top, which creates the space and the freedom for her hair to be simpler to shape and style. It also gives her many styling options; this cut could be made messy and undone, smooth and sleek, or even spiked into a punk-rock look. This is a great all-round style for those that may have hair that is thick enough to make it difficult to manage if the cut is not right.

Modern Mid-Lengths

The Shaggy Freestyle

This is such a fun style to cut and to wear; a similar look should be in every professional's arsenal. A shaggy, featherweight style, being loose and free it plays into the naturally wavy texture of the model's hair. Technically, it can be considered a square layer cut; in realization it is an intuitive cut using the razor to free up the hair into a flowing, soft and contemporary, easy-to-wear style. Notice how length was kept around the face. By draping off the cheekbones, it helps to slim down and frame her features. One of the best things about this cut is that, with a fine and wavy texture, finding a shape that holds its structure is often a challenge, but this style is so soft, playful, and easy that such concerns are irrelevant. Again, this highlights how an experienced pro is able to tailor the shape to the needs of the hair, while enhancing beauty (**Figure 6-8**).

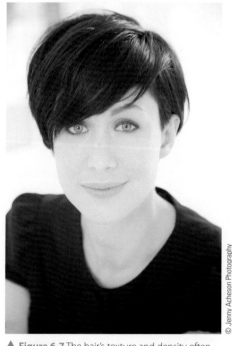

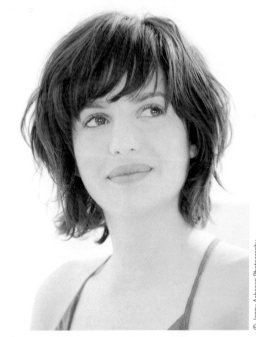

▲ **Figure 6-7** The hair's texture and density often influences the shapes and styles that will be most suitable.

▲ **Figure 6-8** The epitome of a "wash and wear" hairstyle.

Asymmetrical Razor Bob

A classic graduated razor bob cut with the addition of a soft asymmetrical line is a signature style of contemporary razor cutting, and this model is a perfect fit for such a shape. Her naturally red hair is quite thick and coarse, yet this cut creates looseness, swing, and movement for a hair type that might otherwise be weighed down by the heavy density. Razored to just below the jaw to create a strong face frame, the bangs are heavily texturized into a softly separated shape that drapes gracefully over the eye, making this a chic and timeless style. By using the razor to remove length and weight at the same time, the back section blends together with no weight line. It is artistically beautiful and technically perfect (**Figures 6-9 and 6-10**).

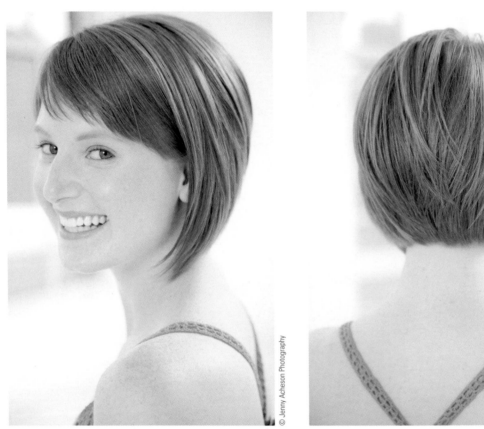

▲ **Figure 6-9 and Figure 6-10** Asymmetry and graduation, cut with a razor, is a great way to put modern swing and movement into bob lengths.

Curl-Enhancing Rounded Layers

Who says the razor cannot cut curls! Evidently, this model has full and bouncy curls full of personality and volume—and the style is cut exclusively with the razor. Natural texture is so unique and beautiful, but the issue here is that there are so many corkscrews and the hair is also so dense and thick that the hair can become easily tangled and hard to control, if the right style choice is not made. Conversely, pick the right style to let those natural curls be the star and handling hair textures like this can produce some of the most aesthetically pleasing results for the client and the stylist. Here the hair was shaped into a heavily layered, rounded razor cut, using a closed-blade technique to create the structure that would hold the shape. Then, to create enough space for the curls to spring to life and prevent tangles, the tipping technique was used to create more room on the interior of the cut (**Figure 6-11**).

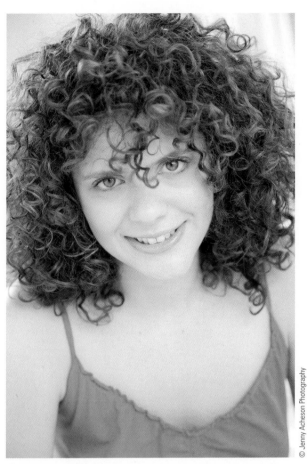

▲ **Figure 6-11** Celebrate natural curls by giving them the space to spring into life.

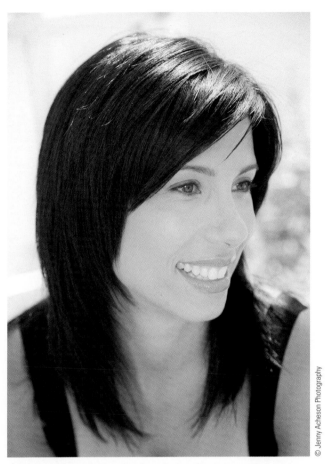

▲ **Figure 6-12** A classic salon-friendly, long layered cut will always be one of the most desirable looks, making it an essential skill for stylists.

Looks for Longer Lengths

Layers and a Side Part

Shiny, smooth, long, and healthy, this hair type is great for stylists to work with, as it presents many options. Unlike definitely thick, fine, or curly hair, where the stylist will probably have certain parameters to work in to create a functional yet fabulous look, here the stylist has more creative freedom, since almost any style will work. A long layered shape with side-parted bangs, this is a simple yet sophisticated style, adding youthfulness and beauty in a polished and easy-to-wear way. The shape also encourages versatile styling options. A round brush blowdry or a few runs with a flat iron creates this sleek look. Alternatively, a few twirls of a curling iron or wand will create a flirty, flowing wave cascade. Make sure you share these styling options with your clients; they will thank you for your professional insight and expertise (**Figure 6-12**).

Long One Length with a Curved Line

This amazing silver-gray color is all natural. Like most gray hair, the texture is coarse. On this occasion, with the dramatic beauty of the hue, a strong one-length curved line complemented by full bangs is the perfect shape. The thickness and the tone of her gray hair is really quite remarkable, and the one-length

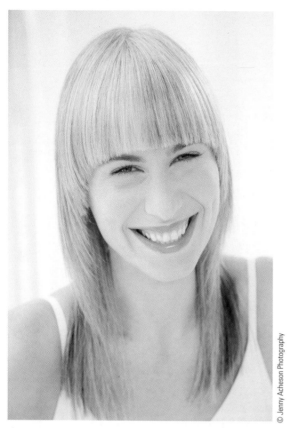

▲ **Figure 6-13** One-length cuts can be strong, powerful, and dramatic.

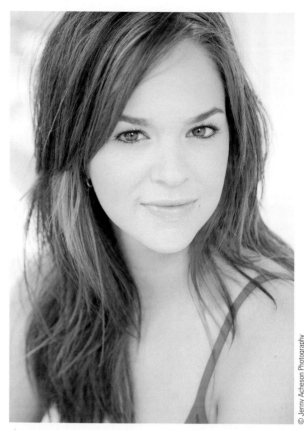

▲ **Figure 6-14** Make your clients look and feel sexy, and fast-track your journey to success.

cut with curve enhances its visual impact (**Figure 6-13**). Instead of softening the coarse density of the hair, as one usually might, one-length lines with full bangs makes her dramatic natural color and texture the star of the style. This highlights the importance of the artistic eye of the hairdresser to be able to see the potential of tailoring a cut to the unique features of each client.

Bombshell Long

This model's hair has a pretty, natural wave and is also thick, long, and luscious. That is an enviable texture, but if the shape of the cut is not right, there is plenty of potential for it to get weighed down into a heavy and unflattering look. To avoid such problems, I razor cut long and loose layers to give natural softness and movement, while maintaining length. The benefit is that it opens the face frame, slims down the features, and creates space for flowing waves to tumble down the neck and shoulders. Given the model's sultry eyes, long and sexy sweeping bangs that drift across the eye line was an easy choice. This is another style made even better because of the versatile styling options. With a paddle brush, a blowdryer, and a smoothing oil or serum, a polished straight look would be as easy to create as these alluring, bombshell waves (**Figure 6-14**).

WHERE YOU GO FROM HERE

Back to class! A joke rooted in truth. As this book testifies, as the styles above show, there is more for you to learn. Obtaining your cosmetology license is not the end of your education, it is the beginning (**Figure 6-15**). Once you finish school, there is nobody to motivate you but you. It is vital to have strong focus, plenty of ambition, and to strive to be the absolute best you can be. Be prepared to work hard and to take ownership of your career and future. Although there are other career paths for cosmetologists, most start by working in a salon. I recommend you consider the first couple of years in the salon as your *advanced apprenticeship*. Being a hairdresser is not a get-rich-quick scheme; it takes time and experience to perfect your techniques and to build confidence and a client base. With this in mind, do not focus on getting behind the chair in a salon right away; focus instead on finding a workplace that has a commitment to stylist education and top-class service. Once you get the skills, you can pay the bills, and have plenty to spend *and* put away.

For now, absorb everything you can from the people around you, take all the education you can get your hands on, and look out for more experienced stylists that can inspire and mentor you. For anyone energized by this supplement book, and who wants to continue their razor cutting journey, make sure your places of work also promote and practice razor cutting.

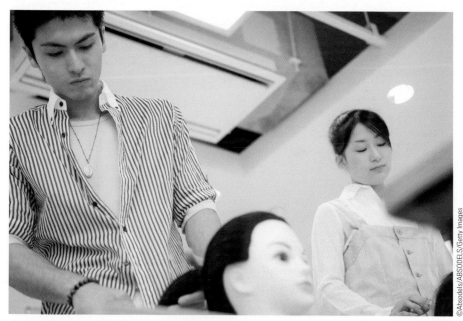

▲ **Figure 6-15** To make career dreams become career reality, vow to never stop learning.

AND FINALLY . . .

Do not let anybody tell you that hairdressing is anything but a high-end career. It is highly creative, independent, and recession proof—people will always need a haircut. The magic of a beauty makeover cannot be outsourced, so you will always have a livelihood. Client-styling in the salon is a great option, and once you build your client base, a six-figure salary is easily attainable. But remember what many forget: Being a salon stylist is not the only option, and it certainly does not need to be the limit of your ambition. You can work in education, in fashion, or in editorial, as well as work as a hairstylist for film, TV, or theatre. In my career I have traveled all over the world, and I get to do things like cover shoots, international shows and seminars, TV and press—as well as run my own hair salon, cosmetology school, advanced education business, and professional product line. The most successful stylists have many strings to their bow. Enjoy your rich and varied life doing the best job in the world (**Figure 6-16**).

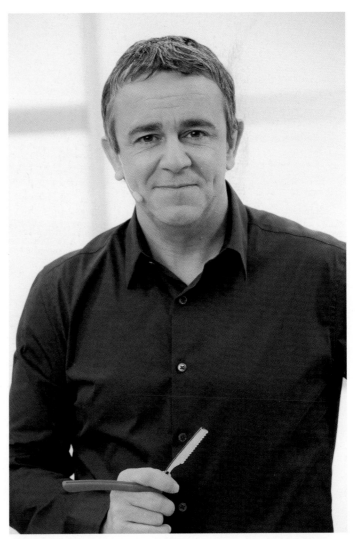

▲ **Figure 6-16** Hairdressing is the best and the happiest job in the world!